Natural Healing Encyclopedia

By Janice McCall Failes and Frank W. Cawood

  FC&A Publishing
  103 Clover Green
  Peachtree City, Georgia 30269

First edition. Printed and bound by the Banta Company. Cover design by Kip Marshall.

ISBN 0-915099-09-8

Acknowledgments

This book is the result of the concern, love and talent of many people. We extend our thanks and gratitude to you.

To all the staff members who contributed their treasured healing secrets: Billie Anderson, Wendy Baas, Audrey Cortez, Sandi Fiveash, Mickey Gore, Anne Joyner, Barbara McMillan, Lois Parker, Linda Sciullo, Mickey Thaxton, Marcia Ulery, and Debbie Williams.

To Linda Sciullo, for your conscientious proofreading and forgiving patience.

To Betty Whitfield, for your superb editing and thoughtful suggestions.

To Kip Marshall, for your art work and design.

To all the staff of FC&A, for your support and willingness to help.

To our spouses, Gayle and B., for your constant encouragement and abiding love.

But, most of all, our thanks and praise is to our Lord and Savior, who created us, heals us and gives us eternal life.

... For we are the temple of the living God;
as God has said,
"I will live in them and move among them,
and I will be their God,
and they shall be my people ...
Since we have these promises, beloved,
let us cleanse ourselves from every defilement
of body and spirit, and make holiness perfect in the
fear of God.
— II Corinthians 6:16b, 7:1
Revised Standard Version

Do you not know that your body is the temple —
the very sanctuary — of the Holy Spirit who lives
within you, Whom you have received (as a gift)
from God? You are not your own, Your were
bought for a price — purchased with a precious-
ness and paid for, made His own. So then, honor
God and bring glory to Him in your body.
— I Corinthians 6:19-20
Amplified Bible

Table of Contents

Introduction

While writing this book, we have discovered many natural ways to help restore your health. Some of these secrets of natural healing have been known for many years, others are newly discovered.

Have you ever wondered why some people are almost never sick? Why one person may look and feel 10 or 20 years younger than his age, while another person the same age may look and feel much older than his age? Many of these healthy people know secrets of natural healing.

This new book, "<u>Natural</u> <u>Healing</u> <u>Encyclopedia</u>", reveals hundreds of natural healing secrets. It shows you how to relieve or prevent many health problems.

The book also mentions certain standard medical treatments. Medical treatment shouldn't be ignored, but natural prevention or treatment may help, too. Natural healing methods which work are a good alternative if your doctor agrees, because they may avoid unpleasant side effects of certain medical treatments.

What Works And What Doesn't Work

The health secrets in this book are not guaranteed to succeed with everyone. As we wrote this book, we realized that we could not pass judgment on the effectiveness of most health secrets that we discovered. Some of these secrets may work for you but not for other people. Some may work for other people but not for you. Many of the health secrets reported in this book may be controversial or unproven by controlled scientific studies. We've simply reported the ideas in this book, because there is some evidence that they have worked for some people. In doing this, we have attempted to separate fact from fiction and to give special attention to natural healing secrets which have been confirmed by scientific research. We have attempted, wherever possible, to verify the accuracy of information reported in this book. Nevertheless, since these are reports of the research of other people, we cannot guarantee their safety or effectiveness.

Because of the possibility of errors in reporting the research of others, and because medical science is such a rapidly expanding field with new developments reported each day, we ask that you consult carefully with your own physician before trying any of the natural healing secrets listed in this book.

It can be dangerous to rely on self-treatment or home remedies and neglect proven medical treatments, such as surgery in cases of cancer. A good physician is the best judge of what sort of medical treatment may be needed for certain diseases. It's good to choose a physician who is open-minded about safe, natural methods of prevention and treatment.

Allergy Relief: See **Asthma** or **Food Allergies**

Alzheimer's Disease

Alzheimer's disease is a progressive deterioration of the brain which can make people unable to care for themselves, cause a loss of memory, loss of ability to solve problems or learn new things, create confusion and cause irritability. It often changes personality, creates an inability to concentrate, and leads to death.

Lecithin supplements may help reduce the risk of developing Alzheimer's. Researchers have found that patients with Alzheimer's disease have a deficiency of acetylcholine in their brain tissue. Acetylcholine is a natural substance that helps transmit nerve reactions in the brain. However, science does not currently know how to replace the lost acetylcholine. Lecithin, a substance extracted from egg yolks, soybeans and other high-fat foods, is thought to be important in replacing acetylcholine. The vitamin choline forms part of the nervous system transmitter acetylcholine and is naturally found in lecithin, soybeans, eggs, fish, liver, wheat germ, green vegetables, peanuts, brewer's yeast, and sunflower seeds.

Memory loss improved in middle-aged people after taking lecithin supplements in a West German study. In a study in England, the progress of Alzheimer's disease was slowed down when lecithin was taken for at least six months. Lipton® soup is hoping to capitalize on these new studies. They are planning to sell a new "healthy" soup containing 80% pure lecithin.

Because Alzheimer's is presently incurable, prevention is especially important. First, don't smoke. A recent study by Stuart Shalat of Harvard University linked cigarette smoking to an increased occurrence of Alzheimer's disease. Based on the study results, people who smoked more than one pack of cigarettes per day were four times as likely to develop Alzheimer's disease as non-smokers, Shalat found.

Avoiding aluminum may help. Autopsies of Alzheimer victims have revealed higher than normal levels of aluminum in brain tissue. Theoretically, preventing the accumulation of aluminum in elderly people may slow or prevent the development of the disease, but scientific studies haven't been completed to prove or disprove this theory. If you want to be cautious and avoid possible exposure to aluminum, avoid foods containing aluminum; do not cook apples, tomatoes or sauerkraut in aluminum pots because these highly acidic foods leech out the aluminum from the cookware; don't buy or drink carbonated beverages from aluminum cans; do not store acidic or salty foods in aluminum foil.

Drinking three glasses of skim milk each day and taking fluoride supplements may help prevent the accumulation of aluminum in the brain.

After death, the only sure way to tell if Alzheimer's disease is present is to do an autopsy on the brain. Doctors are now looking for ways to correctly diagnose the presence of Alzheimer's disease in the living. Alzheimer's seems to cause a specific type of damage to the optic nerve in the eyes, according to studies by Dr. Carol A. Miller published in the New England Journal of Medicine. If the nerve damage is caused only by Alzheimer's disease, it may lead to easier diagnosis of the disease prior to death.

Angina Pectoris

Angina pectoris is chest pain that is caused by heart disease. The amount of angina pain experienced is NOT related to the severity of the heart disease, according to a ten-year study by the U.S. Veterans Administration. Therefore, people with only minor angina may be suffering from extensive heart disease.

Severe angina pectoris is often treated with prescription drugs, but this simple suggestion may help relieve some of the pain. A report in Geriatrics (40:23) recommends raising the head of your bed by about 10 inches, so that gravity helps take some of the strain of circulation off your heart.

Cold can worsen angina attacks. In tests, angina attacks can be brought on by placing the hand of an angina patient in a basin of ice water. Angina sufferers should prepare for cold weather or cold situations by dressing warmly and in layers. Protect your face and head especially, since most of your body's heat escapes from the head. You should avoid going out into cold weather and avoid any strenuous activity in the cold.

Arteries, Hardening of: See **Cholesterol**

Arthritis

Electric blankets are an excellent source of heat for relieving stiffness in people with arthritis. An electric blanket provides consistent, even heat without the bulk of heavy comforters or quilts. Heavy blankets can put too much strain on the feet and joints and cause an arthritis flare-up. Hot water bottles lose their heat too quickly, and heating pads can burn the skin; so an electric blanket may be the best remedy for sore joints.

Some people claim that sleeping in a sleeping bag reduces their morning stiffness. No one is exactly sure why a sleeping bag helps, but it is worth a try if morning stiffness is a problem.

Cold therapy may reduce arthritis pain. Arthritis symptoms sometimes respond well to cold treatments with compresses or ice packs which can serve to reduce inflammation. The Journal of the American Medical Association (JAMA 246: 317) reports that ice cube therapy provided relief for arthritics at Oregon University. For twenty minutes, three times each day, six ice cubes in plastic bags were placed just above and just below the knees of arthritic patients. Even though the cold therapy took a little while to get used to, each patient decided to continue with the ice cube treatment because of the great relief it provided.

To prevent harming the skin by directly applying ice, some doctors recommend making an ice pack from a towel: Soak a small towel in water, then wring it out. Place the towel on a sheet of aluminum foil in a freezer to keep it from sticking to the freezer shelf. Use the towel when ice crystals appear on it, but before it is completely frozen. This "ice pack" will conform to your joints and provide a great cold treatment. Alternating warm and cold sources on the affected area is known to help some arthritic sufferers.

Aspirin has long been recommended as the preferred drug for treatment of the pain and inflammation of arthritis. Now an analog of the active ingredient in aspirin, called salicylate, is found in rub-on creams. For small areas of discomfort using a cream may provide more direct relief. The creams are available over-the-counter as Myoflex® and Aspercreme®. Use them only as directed. If you are allergic to aspirin or if you should not use aspirin because of blood clotting problems, avoid these products.

Support from family, friends and doctors can make a big difference in the pain the patient feels, according to a recent study by researchers at Indiana University. People with osteoarthritis felt better after receiving a phone call from their doctor every two weeks for six months, the researchers discovered. Each phone call lasted about 10 minutes and included questions about how they were feeling and what things they could do for themselves. After the six months, the patients felt less pain than at the beginning of the study. The researchers concluded that although telephone follow-up from doctors could not cure the arthritis, the calls provided emotional support and information for each arthritis sufferer. The calls seemed to relieve the minds of the patients, and they felt less pain, functioned better each day, and were less depressed about their arthritis.

Dr. Arnold Fox of the University of California at Irvine claims that an amino acid can reduce pain in about 80 percent of the general population. The amino acid, DLPA, short for d, l, phenylalanine, is available in many health food stores and drugstores. Dr. Fox recommends 375 to 400 milligrams of DLPA with each meal to reduce the pain of arthritis. DLPA has no known side effects and seems to work by stimulating the body's hormones to block the pain signals from the brain, according to the doctor.

Fish oil supplements may be helpful in reducing morning stiffness and tender joints associated with rheumatoid arthritis, based on a study at Albany Medical College. Nutritionists, however, are recommending incorporating more fish into your regular diet, by eating fish at least twice a week, rather than taking concentrated supplements in capsules or tablets. Salmon, mackerel, tuna, sardines, crab, shrimp, lobster and other shellfish are all high in beneficial omega-3 fatty acids.

Hypnosis may be useful in treating the symptoms associated with arthritis, according to studies by Barbara Domangue, Ph.D. at Jefferson Medical College in Philadelphia. Hypnosis reduced the patients' pain, distress, anxiety and depression and increased the amount of natural painkiller, beta-endorphin, in their blood. Do NOT attempt self-hypnosis, but you may want to discuss the hypnosis option with your doctor or therapist.

Try eliminating some foods from your diet. Some cases of arthritis are caused by allergies according to the medical journal Arthritis and Rheumatism (29:220). A recent case involved a 52-year old woman who displayed symptoms of rheumatoid arthritis only when she drank or consumed milk. To prove the allergy theory, the doctors gave her tablets that she thought were medication on several different occasions. Sometimes the tablets contained a useless substance and sometimes they actually contained powered milk. In each instance, the pain, stiffness, and swelling returned when the woman received the milk, even though the woman did not know what she had been given. This case gives a medical basis for considering allergies in cases of arthritis. If a food allergy is suspected, a rotation diet may help. Also see: **Food Allergies.**

Asthma

Asthma is a chronic but reversible obstruction of the airways affecting about 9 million Americans.

In an asthma attack the airway is narrowed, and the asthmatic struggles to breathe.

Asthma can be disabling and occasionally fatal.

To help prevent asthma attacks, avoid quick or drastic changes in heat or cold or vigorous exercise.

Vitamin A may help in the treatment of bronchial asthma and emphysema. The mineral manganese may reduce allergic reactions in cases of asthma. Vitamin C supplementation is reported to cut allergic and asthmatic attacks in half, according to a controlled scientific study.

Pyridoxine (vitamin B6) may relieve symptoms of asthma and reduce the frequency, duration and severity of asthmatic attacks. Dr. Robert Reynolds, a U.S. Department of Agriculture research chemist, has reported that symptoms "were relieved in every asthmatic tested" when they received 50 milligrams of pyridoxine twice a day. Most patients in the study did not notice an improvement in their asthmatic symptoms until they had taken pyridoxine for four weeks. The best way to treat allergic asthma is to avoid the allergens that trigger the attacks. The home and work environments need to be thoroughly examined. All possible allergens should be avoided if they trigger an attack: pollen, mold, animal hairs, house dust, coal dust, chalk dust, fumes from paints, spray deodorants, varnishes and household cleaners, strong odors including perfume, insecticides, chemicals, tobacco smoke, prescription and over-the-counter drugs, air pollutants, vigorous exercise, and emotional stress.

Strong odors should be avoided, because they can trigger an asthma attack, according to the American Journal of Medicine. Fresh paint, perfumes, tobacco smoke, and cleaning products can all reduce the ability of the lungs to function and trigger an attack in an asthmatic person, says the journal.

Many factors in the workplace can cause asthma including: allergies to grain dust, red cedar wood, and substances used to make plastics. From 5 to 15% of asthma cases are thought to be of occupational origin, giving some types of asthma the nickname "occupational asthma".

Baker's asthma, meat wrapper's asthma and woodworker's asthma are examples.

Sulfites have often been used to preserve fresh food in salad bars, restaurants or in produce sections of grocery stores. Sulfites can cause severe reactions in asthmatics or in non-asthmatics. The FDA knows of seven deaths since October 1982 that may have been caused by sulfites in food. In 1986, the FDA banned the use of sulfites in foods to help protect asthmatics and other sensitive individuals.

Some asthmatics have claimed that coffee provides relief during an asthmatic attack. A recent study in New England Journal of Medicine (310: 743) reports that theobromine, a chemical naturally found in cocoa and also in coffee in smaller quantities, is closely related to the drug theophylline found in tea. Theophylline is often prescribed to treat asthma. The journal suggests that two cups of coffee may provide relief for asthmatics weighing between 100 and 125 lbs. (the amount of the theobromine needed would depend on the size of the patient). However, if asthma patients are taking theophylline and drink coffee as well, they will often experience severe side effects because of the combination.

Doctors at the Milton S. Hershey Medical Center in Pennsylvania discovered that eating aged cheddar cheese can help improve some cases of asthma. The doctors tested the theory at the suggestion of one of their patients who claimed eating cheddar cheese helped relieve his asthma.

Athlete's Foot

Athlete's foot, technically called tinea pedis, is a fungus infection that produces redness and itching between the toes and sometimes elsewhere on the foot. It is quite contagious and can be caught in any public place where bare feet are common.

To help relieve athlete's foot, wash the feet and toes twice a day with plain soap and water, dry thoroughly and change socks. Some people recommend applying honey between the toes two or three times each day. The acid in the honey draws the moisture out of the fungus cells. However, the honey could create a damp breeding ground for more athlete's foot fungus. The best treatment for treating athlete's foot is an over-the-counter antifungus medicine like Desenex® or Tinactin®. Use as directed.

To avoid catching athlete's foot: use rubber

thongs, sandals or plastic bags on your feet when you are taking a shower in a public place; never walk barefoot in a hotel room, athletic locker room, public shower, swimming pool area, or other public place with carpet or plain flooring. Be sure to completely dry your feet, especially in between the toes, after any exposure to water. Change your socks at least once daily or after every activity where your feet have become sweaty, and walk barefoot or wear open sandals without socks as much as possible as the air will allow the feet to dry. When wearing socks, use lightweight cotton socks because they allow better air flow to the feet, and the sweat will evaporate. Change your socks twice daily. Applying plain talcum powder, baking soda or lamb's wool between the toes after drying may be helpful. Try never to wear the same pair of shoes two days in a row. Alternating shoes will give them more time to dry out and prevent the build-up of foot odors and fungus. Buy and wear leather shoes rather than plastic or synthetic, because leather allows the feet to breathe.

Back Problems
One in five adults complains of low back pain each year. It can be caused by muscle strain, stress, improper footwear, menstruation, pregnancy, or improper sitting, standing and sleeping positions.

Here are some simple remedies to help provide relief if you are already experiencing back pain.

(1) Heat, especially moist heat, is the best therapy for back pain. Soaking a towel in hot or boiling water, then wringing it out and placing it on your back can provide fast relief. But be careful! Don't apply the towel if it is still so hot it could scald you. Unfortunately, the heat from the towel will last for only a few minutes. Try placing a plastic bag over the towel after you have put it on your back. The plastic will help keep the heat in.

(2) Learn how to use your bathtub for hydrotherapy. Twenty-minute baths in warm water, rather than extremely hot water, are best. If the water is too hot, your muscles may go into spasm, and that would defeat the purpose of hydrotherapy. If lying in the tub is painful, try buying an inflatable plastic pillow or full body cushion, with suction cups. Lying on an inflated cushion, an extra thick bath mat, or a thick towel, will help relieve the pressure points on your buttocks, hips and back. Don't stretch out completely flat. Try supporting yourself by bending your knees and keeping your feet flat. Move around. Don't lie in one position for too long.

(3) Learn how to use cold water to treat muscle spasms. Cold water treatment seems to help muscle spasms, rather than the muscle pain and tension that warm water relieves. Soaking a towel in icy-cold

water and laying the towel across the area of spasm may be helpful, but most people find that applying an ice pack directly to the area works best. For small areas, the freezer ice packs made for camping may be a good alternative. With either type of pack, we suggest "double-bagging" the pack so ice water doesn't leak out and create more stress. Some doctors recommend making an ice pack from a towel. Soak a small towel in water, then wring it out. Place the towel on a sheet of aluminum foil in a freezer. Use the towel when it has ice crystals on it, but before it is completely frozen. This "ice pack" will conform to your body and provide a great cold treatment.

(4) Exercise. Even while experiencing back pain, contracting and releasing the muscles in your back and stomach may provide some relief. Proper exercise to strengthen the back and abdominal muscles will help prevent future back problems. Brisk walking for about 2 miles, or 30 minutes, a day helps to build up back muscles. Swimming, if you avoid the butterfly and the breast stroke, is also a good way to exercise your back muscles. Some doctors believe back pain is caused when the back muscles are not stretched enough. They recommend Tae Kwon Do (Korean karate) as exercise because the kicking helps to stretch and strengthen the necessary back muscles. Yoga exercises may also be helpful to work and stretch the back

muscles.

The best way to guard against back pain is to be aware of possible strain while working or resting. When working at a workbench or counter, be sure it is at a height that is comfortable for you. If you can place the palm of your hand in the middle of the counter, without bending over, it is at a proper height for you. Avoid jerky movements; take your time when doing physical labor; try arching your back instead of bending over when you cough or sneeze.

The way you sit can aggravate your back muscles. Be sure to use a firm, comfortable seat and sit back in the chair. Keep your knees bent to help use your legs to support your back. Place your feet on a stool or box so your knees are higher than your hips. This position will help relieve the strain on your back and will improve your circulation. Placing a little pillow at the small of your back may be helpful when traveling for long distances by plane, train or car. Never cross your legs. Change positions and get up and move around at least once an hour, if you are usually sitting for a long period of time. Do not remain in a seated position when back pain occurs. Get up and stretch, or lie down for a few minutes before the pain becomes unbearable.

Many people find the new "Swedish-style" back chairs a good alternative to sitting at a desk. In these chairs, you kneel on your knees and sit on a small seat, but the back is not supported. However, the positioning of the chair helps the back to support itself with correct posture. If you have weak back muscles, you might want to try the chair for short periods of time at first, maybe just 15 minutes each day. Then work up gradually to using the chair for all of your desk or typing time.

If you stand for long periods of time, try alternating your weight from foot to foot, or elevate one foot, then the other. We have been taught to place our weight evenly on the balls of both feet; but to prevent back problems, avoid being in one constant position. Be sure to tuck your rear in and don't lock your knees. Keeping the knees slightly bent will also help relieve back strain. When doing dishes or other standing chores, try opening the cupboard door under the sink and putting one of your feet on the ledge at the bottom of the cupboard. This will stop you from locking your knees and will reduce the stress on your back. Slightly raising one leg to relieve back pressure is the idea behind the railing in a bar or pub.

Sleep on a firm mattress, or place a piece of plywood under your mattress for more support. Sleep on your side with your knees bent when possible. When lying on your back, prop up your knees with a pillow or a cushion. Never sleep on your stomach. If you are traveling and sleeping away from your own bed, try taking a piece of plywood with you to place under the mattress, or have someone move the mattress off the box springs and place it on the floor for a better night's sleep.

Learn and use proper lifting techniques. Always use the legs to do the lifting, and bend from the knees, not at the waist. Concentrate on using your thigh muscles, not your back muscles. Never twist while lifting. Keep the object you are lifting as close to your body as you can. When possible, slide objects instead of lifting them. Improper lifting causes most back injuries and leads to the majority of chronic back problems. If you know that your back is sensitive to injury, don't be afraid to ask someone else to lift or move a heavy object for you.

Even when you are carrying everyday items, think about your back. For instance, try carrying a smaller purse; ask the grocery store clerks to put fewer groceries in each bag, so they aren't as heavy to carry.

Buy shoes that will help support you properly. Many women with back problems have discovered that just by wearing low-heeled shoes (1/2" high or lower) they have eliminated their back problems. It isn't always so simple, but proper footware (shoes that help your back support your weight) is important. Dressing properly, like carrying an extra sweater or coat, could also prevent chills and unnecessary back muscle aggravation.

Arch supports may help relieve back pain even if

you are not flat-footed, according to research at Hillel Jaffe Hospital in Hadera, Israel. The way the heel of the foot hits the ground can cause a disturbing shock to your spine and aggravate your back. In the study in Israel sixty percent of the patients found the arch supports relieved their back pain in just three to four weeks. Ninety percent of the participants found the arch supports effective within a year.

Wear loose and comfortable clothing. Many children complaining of lower back pain have been wearing jeans that were too tight. Heavy jeans with reinforced seams can cause back problems. If possible, avoid wearing jeans, or wear loose-fitting jeans.

Lose weight. Chiropractor, Dr. Alan J. Lichter of Washington, D. C. says "every extra pound on your stomach puts 10 pounds more stress on your low back". Think of how much strain lifting a 20 pound sack of potatoes would put on your back, then realize that, if you are 20 pounds overweight, this forces your back to carry many of those extra pounds. Proper nutrition and good eating habits will help you lose weight and improve your overall health. After big meals, like Thanksgiving, Christmas or other special occasions, Dr. Lichter recommends a 15-20 minute walk to relieve possible back discomfort and speed the use of extra calories.

Bad Breath

Bad breath (medically known as halitosis) frequently originates in the mouth. It can be caused by poor dental hygiene, food stuck between the teeth, dental plaque, inflamed gums, or food stuck in the gums. Proper brushing after every meal or snack, daily flossing, brushing the tongue and regular visits to the dentist can help eliminate bad breath caused by poor dental hygiene.

Bad breath can also be caused by illnesses that affect the entire body, like liver or kidney failure, or diabetes. In these cases, the illness must be treated to help eliminate the cause of the bad breath.

However, older people with good dental hygiene and no overall illnesses may still suffer from bad breath, the Journal of the American Medical Association (JAMA 254: 2473) reports. Sometimes this bad breath is caused by a dry mouth or lack of saliva. In cases of dryness, mucus may be crusting and allowing bacteria to grow in the mouth and nose. Drinking plenty of water and using a humidifier will help combat bad breath problems caused by dryness.

Eating parsley is claimed to help sweeten your breath naturally.

Bed Sores: See Pressure Sores

Bee Stings: See **Insect Bites And Stings**

Birthmarks
<u>The</u> <u>Archives</u> <u>of</u> <u>Dermatology</u> reports that the best method for treating the reddish-purple birth marks (called Port Wine Stains) is a new laser treatment using a pulsed yellow-dye laser. This special laser treatment, developed by Dr. Oon Tian Tan at Boston University School of Medicine, may replace the traditional laser therapy that sometimes damages the outer layer of skin when removing Port Wine Stain birthmarks.

Bites: See **Insect Bites And Stings**

Blisters
Blisters, caused by friction, can be very painful and require special care and attention. The best treatment for a blister is to gently wash the unbroken blister with soap and water and cover the whole area with a bandage.

Do NOT break a blister unless it is on the foot or some other place that will be exposed to continued friction. If breaking the blister is necessary, wash the unbroken blister and the surrounding area thoroughly. Then, take a sterilized needle and gently prick the blister. Squeeze the fluid out gently and carefully, and cover the entire area with a bandage. Do NOT remove any skin, because the flap of skin will help protect the area and speed the recovery time.

While a blister is healing, try to protect it from any further rubbing or friction. Cover the area of the blister with a bandage or moleskin to allow it time to heal. If you know your shoes or boots are causing friction, tape the area of friction before participating in any activity. If you can feel a "hot spot" that you think will develop into a blister, protect it right away. The longer you leave it, the more painful it will become.

To prevent foot blisters, be sure that your socks fit your feet properly, and that they are not folded inside your shoes or boots. Socks that are too large and cause bagging can cause blisters. Try wearing two pairs of very thin socks, rather than one thicker pair. Friction will occur between the socks, and your feet will be protected. Be careful to buy shoes that fit properly. Take time to "break in" new shoes by wearing them on carpet for just a few minutes at a time. Gradually build-up your time until the shoes are comfortable.

Blood Clots

Crossing the legs may be the most common reason that women suffer from blood clots. Crossing the legs impairs the flow of blood in the veins and arteries of the legs. Especially when varicose veins or vascular disease is present, the slower blood flow may cause formation of blood clots. Clots can be deadly if they move to your lungs, heart or brain. Since women have been taught to tightly cross their legs to be lady-like, it is a very difficult habit to break, but it is worth the effort. Crossing your legs at the ankles is not as harmful but should also be avoided if possible.

Sitting for long periods of time while recuperating from illness, traveling or working can also lead to formation of blood clots. Be sure to get up and walk around at least once every two hours to renew the circulation to your legs and feet. Wiggle your feet and ankles whenever possible to improve circulation.

Blood clots can be a serious problem after surgery, but some non-drug methods can help keep them from occurring in the legs, according to research at the Northwestern University Medical School. The surgeons there recommend wearing thigh-length elastic hose (called anti-embolism stockings) for at least three days prior to surgery, and wearing inflatable tubular sleeves (called long leg compression devices) for at least three days after surgery. Both the sleeves and the hose provide external compression on the legs, which helps to prevent blood clots, without the risk of other complications.

Blood Pressure — High

Daily breathing exercises may help reduce high blood pressure. Practice by lying flat on your back on a carpeted floor. Prop up your head, and put a cushion under your knees so you are completely comfortable and relaxed. Breathe in slowly (to the count of ten), hold for 2 seconds, then breathe out slowly (another count of ten). Many people feel that they are practicing good breathing just by breathing in slowly, but slow exhaling is just as important. By doing these deep breathing exercises for only 3 to 5 minutes each day, you will feel relaxed and may lower your blood pressure and pulse rate.

Black licorice or licorice extracts should be avoided if you suffer from high blood pressure, according to researchers at Tufts University. Black licorice can make the body hold onto sodium (salt), lose potassium and cause fluid retention. People taking diuretics for their high blood pressure should be especially careful to avoid licorice, because it seems to compound the problems and bad side effects of the diuretic drugs. About 90% of the licorice imported into the United States is used in chewing tobacco; this is one of many reasons people with high blood pressure should avoid all forms of tobacco.

Avoid holding your breath when straining, according to <u>Cardiac</u> <u>Alert</u> newsletter. This "Valsalva Maneuver" counteracts the natural tendency to hold your breath when you are trying to lift, pull, push or move something during a bowel movement or while exercising. Many times, people hold their breath and grunt and groan when straining. However, holding your breath during these strenuous times causes your blood pressure to skyrocket and puts additional pressure on your heart and arteries. Practice breathing in and out slowly and steadily. Consciously breathe during any strenuous activity.

Then, when lifting or moving something make sure you have enough people or support to properly move the object. (Avoid all straining during bowel movements — as well as increasing your blood pressure, the strain may cause hemorrhoids and bowel problems. High fiber diets help people avoid straining at stool.)

The disposition of your spouse and your partner's blood pressure level have a great influence on your blood pressure. At the University of Texas, Marjorie A. Speers, Ph.D. discovered the relationship after examining over 1,200 couples. Other factors, like exercise, salt intake and obesity were taken into consideration, but the spouse still influenced the blood pressure levels. Perhaps a program for both the husband and the wife, including health care and counseling, could help in this situation.

Although the doctor may never say, "Take one puppy and call me in the morning", many health professionals are now recommending the loving companionship and responsibility that a pet provides. According to medical studies, in some cases pets can help people reduce their high blood pressure levels. Pets can help people to relax and feel loved. Almost half of the psychologists, psychiatrists and family doctors that participated in a recent survey have prescribed "pet therapy" for emotional problems like depression and loneliness. Since emotional problems can contribute to high blood pressure, pets may play an important role in therapy. Many doctors and therapists feel that pets provide love, support, an opportunity for exercise and a reason for living. If tension is contributing to a person's blood pressure problems, a pet may provide the relaxation needed. A recent study has shown that elderly people with pets lived longer than those without these little companions.

Blood Pressure — Low

People with low blood pressure often have difficulty standing up quickly. Because their bodies cannot quickly supply enough blood to the brain, they suffer from dizziness, fainting, light-headedness, blurred vision and shaking. Just as high blood pressure causes problems to the whole body, low blood pressure can be very dangerous.

Researchers at Vanderbilt University Medical Center in Nashville claim that coffee can help raise blood pressure that is too low. Many older people have trouble with low blood pressure, dizziness, fainting, or even collapsing after eating a large breakfast. Two cups of coffee in the morning seem to help combat all these symptoms. However, according to New England Journal of Medicine, for the coffee to be effective in the morning, it must be completely avoided for the rest of the day.

Body Odor

Nurses at Veterans Administration Hospital in Colorado have discovered that a favorite pet remedy is also good for human beings. Rural families have known for years that if an animal is sprayed by a skunk that washing in tomato juice gets rid of the odor. To relieve body odor, anyone can soak for 15 minutes in a tub of water, with about 24 ounces of tomato juice and a few drops of mineral oil. The mineral oil helps to balance the acid of the tomato juice and keeps the skin from drying out. This method was also used by nurses in World War

I to help eliminate odors from patients suffering with gangrene, says the <u>American</u> <u>Journal</u> <u>of</u> <u>Nursing</u>.

Breast Disease — Fibrocystic

About 20 percent of women between 25 and 50 years of age are thought to have fibrocystic breast disease. This disease produces non-cancerous breast lumps that cause soreness, swelling and pain in women, with the symptoms usually appearing just prior to monthly menstruation.

Many doctors are recommending elimination of caffeine and similar chemicals called methylxanthines to help relieve fibrocystic breast disease. Caffeine is found in coffee, tea, cola and pepper drinks, chocolate, and some prescription and over-the-counter drugs. However, in a recent article in the <u>Archives</u> <u>of</u> <u>Internal</u> <u>Medicine</u>, Drs. Wendy Levinson and Patrick Dunn at Good Samaritan Hospital in Portland, Oregon claim that there isn't any "good evidence" linking caffeine and fibrocystic breast disease. Levinson and Dunn reviewed all the previous medical studies linking caffeine and fibrocystic breast disease and do not think that women should routinely give up caffeine because of the fibrocystic disease.

Vitamin E has been used to reduce the non-cancerous swellings found in fibrocystic breast disease. Dr. Robert London of Baltimore discovered that 600 I.U.'s of vitamin E each day is helpful in reducing the disease in about 70 percent of affected women.

Breasts (Sore Breasts Due To Nursing)

Many doctors are now applying vitamin E drops directly onto the sore and cracked nipples of nursing mothers. There is no scientific evidence that this helps the breasts, but doctors around the country seem to think it helps.

Another (though doubtful) suggestion for nursing mothers is placing wet tea bags on the nipples. This is done in some hospitals to help keep the nipples moist and to avoid the soreness. However, tea contains tannin which is thought to be a cancer-causing agent. Tannin can also stain the skin, so we cannot recommend tea bags as a good remedy.

Bunions

Bunions are a swelling or deformity of the big toe usually caused by improperly-fitting shoes. Most people who suffer from bunions are middle-aged and older women who have worn tight, pointed-toe, high-heeled shoes throughout most of their lives. In countries where high heels are not worn, like Japan where, until recently, sandals were worn, bunions were infrequent. However, some people may be genetically inclined to get bunions.

Once a bunion appears, here are some suggestions to help relieve the pain. Wear only shoes or sandals that do not constrict your big toe and the wide part of your foot (called the toe box). Wear shoes with heels less than two inches high. If necessary, have your shoes widened or stretched by a shoe-repairer.

Small pads, like corn pads, can be made especially for people suffering from bunions. The pads have a hole for the bunion and help to distribute the pressure away from the area of the bunion.

Some exercises to stretch and strengthen the big toe and foot muscles may help alleviate some of the pain and help prevent the bunion from getting worse.

Once a bunion is healed, do NOT go back to wearing tight-fitting, high-heeled shoes. Wearing comfortable shoes or sandals is the only way to help prevent bunions from recurring.

Burns

Raw egg whites applied to simple, non-severe kitchen burns are reported to give fast relief and help the burn to heal.

In badly burned patients, live yeast may help the skin heal faster, says Dr. Jerold Z. Kaplan of

Berkeley, California. Dr. Kaplan tested yeast on skin grafts and burn victims. People treated with the yeast healed faster and developed less scarring than people who did not receive the yeast treatment. Perhaps live yeast treatments, like that found in some hemorrhoid creams, will give help for non-severe kitchen burns.

Calluses: See **Corns Or Calluses**

Cancer

In a recent study, people who didn't drink milk were three times as likely as milk drinkers to get colorectal cancer. The study was conducted by Chicago Western Electric Company, and researchers at the University of California in San Diego interpreted the data. Drinking two or three glasses of skim milk each day may help prevent colorectal cancer, according to this study. It is important to not take vitamin D supplements while drinking lots of vitamin D fortified milk, because of possible overdose of vitamin D, which can be toxic.

Avoiding skin exposure to the sun has been publicized as an important way to reduce your chances of getting skin cancer, but your eyes also need to be protected from the sun's ultraviolet rays. According to the New England Journal of Medicine (13,

313), a deadly cancer of the eye, called intraocular malignant melanoma, is mostly likely to occur in people who have spent a lot of time outdoors, sun bathers or those who use sun lamps. You can lower your risk by wearing protective sun glasses, hats, or visors while in the sun. Sitting under an umbrella at the beach may protect you from direct sunlight, but the dangerous rays bounce off the sand and back under the umbrella. Even under an umbrella, you should still protect your eyes and wear a sunscreen to protect your skin.

Fruits and vegetables may help protect you against certain types of stomach cancer, according to research at the Louisiana State University published in the Journal of the National Cancer Institute (76: 4, 621). Eating crunchy yellow and dark green vegetables, like broccoli, spinach, cauliflower and carrots, has received a lot of attention in the media, but eating other vegetables and fruits can also lower rates of stomach cancer. The study at Louisiana State found people who ate an above-average amount of fruit and vegetables were only HALF as likely to have a precancerous stomach condition called chronic atrophic gastritis. Increasing your intake of all fruit and vegetables is recommended.

Substances found in garlic and onions are now being studied as a possible way to slow down cancer. Dr. Michael Wargovich at the University of Texas has shown that organic sulfides in garlic and onions slow the progress of colon cancers in experiments. Be careful about increasing the amount of garlic and onions that you eat though, eating them in large quantities can have some unpleasant side effects like bad breath.

Women who eat eggs or fried foods die from ovarian cancer at three times the rate of women who avoid those foods, according to research by Dr. David A. Snowden from the University of Minnesota. Dr. Snowden has also discovered an increased risk of prostate cancer in men who eat animal products as compared to men who follow a vegetarian diet. People who drink coffee are at a greater risk of dying from bladder or colon cancer, and male coffee drinkers have an increased risk of death from coronary artery disease, the study concluded.

Having a desk job may increase the risk of getting colon cancer by 30%, according to two recent studies. State University in Buffalo, New York found that men with inactive jobs were twice as likely to get colon cancer compared to men who had active jobs. The Swedish National Institute of Environmental Medicine discovered that men who sat down for more than half of the work day had a 30% higher rate of colon cancer than men who were more physically active on the job. It seems that long periods of sitting allows the body's waste, and the cancer causing substances in it, to collect in the colon for longer periods of time. Extra concern for a proper, high-fiber diet and plenty of exercise should be a top priority for both men and women with desk jobs.

Calcium supplements may reduce the risk of colon cancer, according to research by Dr. Martin Lipkin at the Memorial Sloan-Kettering Cancer Center. In these tests, calcium helped lower precancerous changes in the bowel and may help reduce the occurrence of stomach cancers.

Limit your intake of pickled or cured foods and luncheon meats. Pickled foods contain high amounts of salt, and cured foods often contain nitrites which can turn into cancer-inducing nitrosamines.

Canker Sores

A canker sore is a raw ulcer that is located inside the mouth. Canker sores are not contagious, but they are often painful and periodically affect about one-quarter of the population. They can occur anywhere in the mouth, including under the tongue, on the inside of the cheek or lips, or anywhere on the gums.

Doctors believe that some canker sores are caused by bad dental hygiene, improperly fitting dentures, fevers, tension, overtiredness, using a "hard toothbrush", hormonal changes during menstruation, or allergic reactions to certain foods. Many people get canker sores only after they have eaten specific foods, like citrus fruits, spices, chocolate, nuts, aged cheese, milk, or carbonated drinks containing cola.

There is no standard cure for canker sores. Some doctors recommend gargling with salt water (about 2 teaspoons of salt to one-half cup water). Although this is painful, gargling and swishing with salt water combined with immediate attention to regular brushing and flossing, seem to speed healing.

Dr. R.E. Couch of Watkinsville, Georgia recommends rinsing the mouth, once daily, with a mixture of half 3% hydrogen peroxide solution and half water to quickly heal any mouth sores.

At one time, doctors recommended holding a quarter of an aspirin directly on the canker sore. However, this can damage the sensory nerves in the mouth and should NOT be used.

To prevent canker sores, be sure to brush your teeth after every meal with a soft toothbrush, floss your teeth once a day, have dentures fixed or refitted, take out partial dentures at night, keep partials and full dentures immaculately clean, replace your toothbrush once a month, avoid using mouthwash, strive to get plenty of rest, do not use chewing gum or suck on hard candy or lozenges, and avoid stressful situations. Obviously, if you think your canker sores may be an allergic reaction to a specific food, try avoiding that food. If canker sores do recur, try to determine what you ate that might have caused them.

Cholesterol Reduction

Reducing cholesterol in your blood can lower your risk of having coronary artery disease. According to the Coronary Prevention Trial at the Lipid Research Clinic, each 1% drop in the serum cholesterol level can lower the risk of having a major heart attack by 2%.

Eat chick-peas, soybean products, oats, and carrots to help maintain low cholesterol levels. Oat bran is an excellent source of water-soluble fiber that can reduce blood cholesterol levels from 6 to 19%, based on data from the Lipid Research Clinic.

Researchers at Northwestern University (Journal Of The American Dietetic Association) discovered that about two cups of oatmeal or two oat bran muffins daily, combined with moderate dietary levels of fat and cholesterol, can lower blood cholesterol levels in just a few weeks. If you prefer oat bran muffins, be sure to use a low cholesterol substitute, rather than eggs, in the muffins.

Two fish oils, EPA and DHA known as omega-3 fatty acids, have been proven to help lower serum cholesterol. (New England Journal of Medicine

312: 1205-1209).   Natural fish oils are found in oily, cold-water fish like trout, salmon, tuna, herring, and mackerel, and in other fish in lower concentrations. Unfortunately, canning tuna and salmon destroys most of the important oils. Therefore, it is best to increase the amount of fish in your diet without relying on canned salmon or tuna. Some fish oil supplements are now available for over-the-counter supplementation of omega-3 fatty acids. Fish oil can reduce the blood's ability to clot, so DO NOT take fish oil supplements with aspirin treatment or prior to surgery.

Daily garlic may be good for you by helping to reduce the levels of LDL (low-density lipoprotein) cholesterol in the blood, raising the level of HDL (high-density lipoprotein) cholesterol, therefore lowering the chances of blood clots, according to a study in The American Journal of Clinical Nutrition. The study used specially extracted garlic oil which equalled eating 10 cloves of garlic daily. In six months, the level of HDL cholesterol (the "good" type of cholesterol that can help prevent coronary heart disease) was increased by 41%. However, eating 10 cloves of garlic daily could provide some unwanted side effects like bad breath, diarrhea and body odor. Unfortunately, according to these researchers, the garlic pills, oils and extracts currently sold in health food stores do not contain the necessary ingredients to help in the cholesterol battle.

Try to avoid artificial and non-dairy creamers. If you need to use a powdered product (due to lack of refrigeration) use low-fat powdered milk. It is still convenient but has a lower fat content than a non-dairy cream substitute. Don't use foods containing coconut or palm oil, because they are high in saturated fats.

Cold Sensitivity

Keeping the body at a regular temperature of 98.6°F is very important, especially in elderly people who have lost some of their natural defenses against the cold.

During cold winter months, visit your elderly friends and relatives often to make sure they are not accidentally losing too much body heat. Make sure that there are enough blankets on the bed for sleeping and naps and that the furnace is set between 65 and 70°F. Many older people have lost their ability to shiver, which is a natural protection against cold. Without shivering, they do not realize that the temperature is too cold. Since prescription drugs can inhibit our ability to protect ourselves from the cold, the older folks are once again especially at risk. Medicine for high blood pressure, sedatives, antidepressants and alcohol can all dull the body's perceptions and ability to notice cold.

And since many older people are on limited budgets, they try to save money by keeping the furnace down low and by eating only small meals. Each person should try to get at least one hot, balanced meal each day.

Vitamin C supplementation may help to reduce sensitivity to cold temperatures. Magnesium supplements may aid in adaptation to the cold.

Alcoholic beverages should be avoided in extreme hot or cold temperatures. Extreme temperatures can turn a regular amount of consumed alcohol into a lethal dose. Alcohol hinders temperature regulation of warm-blooded animals according to studies at the University of Southern California's School of Pharmacy. Alcohol, mixed with cold weather or a cold house, can cause a severe loss of body temperature and could possibly lead to death.

To improve circulation and avoid getting too cold, elderly people should also get some exercise every day. Whether it is walking a short distance or rocking in a rocking chair, physical activity is needed to help keep circulation flowing and maintain good body heat. Dr. Arthur Helfand of the Medical Center in Philadelphia says a rocking chair can provide as much exercise as walking. It uses important muscles in the legs and feet and improves circulation. Almost anyone can rock in a rocking chair.

Colds

In treating common colds, chicken soup has been scientifically shown to be more effective than other hot liquids, according to the medical journal, Chest. Chicken soup, especially homemade chicken soup with chicken parts, noodles, herbs and spices, helps to clear mucus from the nose, says the journal. Homemade soup also contains less salt than store-bought varieties, which is another reason why homemade soup is preferred. Drinking it and breathing the steaming air rising from the soup is recommended as the first step in home treatment for coughs and the common cold.

If you have very sticky or thick phlegm in your nose, you will want to help liquefy the mucus so it will clear out more easily when you blow your nose. Drinking plenty of fluids, especially hot soup, and eating hot spicy food, may be helpful. Do not eat or drink any dairy products, like milk, eggs, or cheese, as they cause the mucus to thicken.

Blow your nose gently because blowing your nose with too much power can also force mucus into the ear canals and cause ear infections.

If the inside of the nose is noticeably dry, try rubbing a little bit of petroleum jelly in the nostrils. Sometimes, a dry nose will cause the body to produce too much mucus, which causes a stuffed nose. Petroleum jelly will help keep the nose moist and help regulate the body's mucus production.

Applying petroleum jelly on dry nose tissue may help prevent a cold or shorten the length of a cold.

Dry air contributes towards dry noses and throats. To breathe easier, add moisture to the air, especially in your bedroom, using a humidifier. Breathing warm, moist air, such as in a shower or vapor clouds from a kettle or a hot water vaporizer, only after the steam has cooled and condensed, is also effective. Be careful using hot-water vaporizers or steam kettles because they can cause burns.

Nose drops made of salt and water (1/4 teaspoon of salt added to eight ounces of water) may help to clear the nose and ease breathing.

Try sleeping on an extra pillow so it will be easier for your nasal passages to drain while you are sleeping.

If the lungs are completely congested, making it difficult to breathe, try drinking coffee or other beverage containing caffeine. Caffeine helps to dilate the bronchial tubes which may make breathing a little easier. Theophylline, a caffeine-like drug found in tea, is even more effective than caffeine. Another suggestion is to mix 2 tablespoons of vinegar and 2 tablespoons of honey into one cup of lemon juice. Heat and sip a little of the lemon juice, honey and vinegar combination. Even though it will be difficult to sip, it should help clear your congestion.

Disinfecting your toothbrush can kill the cold-causing germs and prevent you from re-infecting yourself. Try disinfecting your toothbrush by soaking it in a dilute hydrogen peroxide solution, then thoroughly rinsing the toothbrush with water before using it.

Or, rather than trying to disinfect your toothbrush, some dentists recommend throwing it away at the beginning signs of a cold. Then discard the new toothbrush as soon as the cold or throat infection is cleared up. Dr. Tom Glass of the Oklahoma University School of Dentistry discovered that colds, sore throats, gum disease, mouth sores and some other infections keep returning because the organisms are reproducing right on your toothbrush. During any infection in the mouth, Dr. Glass recommends using your toothbrush for only one month. And remember, even when you are completely healthy, the American Dental Association recommends that you replace your toothbrush every three to four months.

Don't stifle a sneeze. A sneeze is the body's natural way to clean out the nose passages to allow easy breathing. Be sure to cover the nose and mouth area during a sneeze, preferably with a handkerchief. But if you try to stifle or "hold back" the sneeze, the phlegm and the cold germs can be forced into the ears. Ear infections, ear noises and recurring colds can be caused or aggravated by stifling sneezes.

To keep your neck warm while fighting off a cold or sore throat, try tying a sock or scarf around your neck. It may look unusual, but as long as you're at home suffering with a cold, it shouldn't matter what you look like, as long as it works!

To keep from spreading colds, wash your hands after wiping your nose and right after contact with a person with a cold. During a cold, flush your used facial tissues down the toilet; if you sneeze, cover your nose and mouth with a facial tissue and wash your hands thoroughly after your sneeze. Do not use the telephone, typewriter, bar of soap, towel, pencil or pen of someone that has a cold. After a cold, be sure to clean these items so you do not re-infect yourself.

Cold Sores: See **Fever Blisters**

Colic

Colic is often described as unexplained crying by a child up to four months of age. Usually the crying occurs at the same time every day or night. Doctors are not exactly sure what causes colic, but here are some natural ways to help deal with this annoying situation, if the baby's doctor determines that crying is caused by colic and nothing more serious.

During a colicky spell, give the baby a bottle with one or two ounces of warm water. Try laying the baby face down in his crib, with a hot water bottle under his stomach. Play soothing, gentle music to provide a relaxed atmosphere for the baby. Rock the child with a gentle motion, or try getting and using a water-bed crib for the baby. The gentle rocking motion of a swing or cradle, or a car ride, often reduces the crying. Playing or any change in scenery, like a walk in a park, may be helpful.

If you are breast-feeding, your diet is important. Try avoiding cow's milk and milk products, chocolate, caffeine, alcohol, broccoli, spicy foods, beans, brussel sprouts, carbonated drinks, melons, apples, wheat flour products and any other foods that can produce gas. If the baby is on a formula, check with your doctor to find an alternative to cow's milk, such as soy milk. Never leave a colicky baby alone with a propped bottle. Always feed the baby in an upright position so he swallows as little air as possible. Burp the baby frequently, during feeding and just after feeding. Try giving the baby smaller feedings more times during the day. More frequent feedings, with less to drink, may help reduce the colic.

A spoonful of calcium gluconate syrup before feedings is sometimes recommended as being helpful for colic.

A colicky baby often requires special patience

from a mother because the constant crying doesn't give the mother adequate rest time. Take time for yourself by having a relative or friend look after the child (or children) for at least a couple of hours every day so you can get some rest. You need to keep yourself in good health so you can deal with the stress of a colicky baby. In some cases, tension in a family may increase the colicky baby's crying, so try to get family members to rest whenever possible.

Constipation

Constipation is a frequently misunderstood term. Medically speaking, it refers to a hard, dry stool which is difficult to pass. Many people think it means not having a bowel movement daily. The National Institutes of Health says that each person requires a slightly different bowel schedule — once a day is normal for some people, but three times a week might be normal for another person.

Regularity should be achieved by completely natural methods: eat foods high in fiber content like whole grain products, fresh fruit, fresh vegetables and unprocessed foods; drink lots of fluids; get plenty of exercise; and take time for your bowel movements. Avoid using commercial laxatives. Frequent use of laxatives can cause constipation, because laxatives make the body's natural bowel movement mechanisms insensitive. If mineral oil is used as a laxative, it can lead to a deficiency of some vitamins, including vitamins A, D, E and K, says <u>Pharmacy Times</u>. Mineral oil doesn't allow the body to properly absorb these vitamins from food.

Coffee may help with regularity, according to a study by researchers at the University of Kansas College of Health Sciences and Hospital. The researchers tested a theory that many of their patients had claimed for years. Without their coffee in the morning, they just couldn't "get going". They discovered that 2-1/2 cups of regular or decaffeinated coffee did produce more frequent and easy bowel movements, compared to drinking other warm beverages or going without coffee. (All the people in the test were placed on identical diets so the amount of fiber, the best source of regularity, did not affect the study results).

In other research, drinking a cup of hot water about half an hour before breakfast seems to have a mild laxative effect. Maybe this is partially why hot coffee is so effective!

For many years, prunes, raisins and figs have been recommended as natural laxatives, presumably only because they are a good source of fiber. However, scientists have recently found that a natural laxative called diphenylisatin is found in prunes.

Corns Or Calluses

Corns are the most common foot problem in older Americans. Corns usually appear on the toes and are the result of undue pressure or friction, usually from improperly-fitting shoes. Calluses are usually flat and wide; corns are usually cone-shaped.

Corns and calluses are actually layers of dead skin. They form at a point where friction or pressure causes the blood supply to that area to be increased. This causes the tissue cells there to grow more rapidly, and an overgrowth of cells occurs.

Corns are more painful than calluses, even though the corn itself is dead skin. When pressure is applied to the corn, it can hit a nerve and be extremely painful. The larger the corn, the more likely it is that it will be painful when external pressure or friction occurs.

The first step to prevent corns and calluses is to wear only shoes or sandals that do not constrict your toes or feet. Wear shoes that have less than two-inch heels, so you don't put extra pressure on your toes. If necessary, have your shoes widened or stretched by a shoe-repairer. Discard or give away any shoes that do not fit you comfortably and properly.

Once a corn or callus appears, you can help relieve the soreness by wearing moleskin around the corn or using a hole-in-the-center corn pad. This will take the pressure off the corn and should help relieve any pain.

To remove the corn or callus, ONLY the DEAD layers of skin should be taken off. Soak your foot in hot water or castor oil for at least 15 minutes. Then gently scrub the dead skin away with an emery board, rough towel or a pumice stone. Scrub off only dead skin and never use a razor or knife to cut off the skin! Stop scrubbing if the area around the corn or callus appears red. Repeat this procedure at least twice a week. Unfortunately, the corn or callus will come back if you don't change your shoes or the pressure that originally created the corn or callus.

If you have diabetes or a circulation problem, you should discuss your corns and calluses with a doctor because home treatment could be dangerous for you.

Coughs

Each year in the United States millions of dollars are spent on cough remedies. Yet many of these over-the-counter remedies do not contain ingredients that are proven to help coughs caused by common colds or the flu. Coughing is a natural reflex that helps keep our breathing passages free of mucus and other secretions. Coughing should not be suppressed when it is helping our body to clean itself of foreign material.

If the cough is dry or irritating, it can prevent you from getting the rest or sleep that you need to help fight the infection. To soothe the throat, sucking a piece of ice is just as effective as most over-the-counter cough drops. Most cough drops contain sugar or corn syrup, which is actually "food" for any bacteria growing in the throat. Drinking warm, clear liquids, like coffee or tea, is an effective way to soothe the throat and ease coughing spells.

If you have very sticky or thick phlegm in your breathing passages, you will want to help liquefy the secretions so they are easier to cough up. Drinking plenty of fluids, especially hot soup, and eating hot spicy food may be helpful. Do not eat or drink any dairy products, like milk or cheese, or eggs because they may cause mucus to thicken. Breathing moist air, like in a shower, clouds of vapor from a kettle, a moist humidifier, or vaporizer, is also effective. Be careful not to breathe hot steam.

If the lungs are completely congested, making it difficult to breathe, try drinking coffee, tea or other beverages containing caffeine. Tea is especially good because it contains theophylline. These drugs help to dilate the bronchial tubes and make breathing a little easier.

Cuts (Lacerations)

Small, minor cuts can easily be treated at home after checking with your doctor. Wash the cut with soap and water. Be sure to get all dirt and foreign objects out of the wound, and clean the area around the wound. Keep the cut clean and then allow the edges of the cut to stay together for proper healing.

Apply ice as soon as possible to reduce swelling and bleeding which can slow healing and lead to scarring. However, if you notice tingling or numbness around the cut or in joints close by, or if you have a very large cut or know that a dirty object caused the cut, you should see your doctor or visit an emergency clinic as soon as possible.

A study in The American Journal of Surgery (145:374) shows that wounds heal faster when unboiled commercial honey is applied directly onto cleaned wounds.

Vitamins and minerals help wounds heal. Vitamin C is essential for the fast healing of wounds and surgical incisions. Taking extra vitamin C before surgery and after an injury is proven to help the healing process. The mineral copper also helps the healing processes of the body.

Zinc is involved in the synthesis of nucleic acid (DNA and RNA) so it is directly related to growth and repair of the body. It helps burns and wounds heal and helps the B vitamins work. Vitamin B12 is essential for cell reproduction, which makes it necessary for bone growth and cell repair.

If you get a cut at the ocean, the seawater will not clean the wound properly. There is a common misperception that seawater heals wounds so that they don't need to be treated. However, seawater contains hundreds of tiny micro-organisms that can cause infections. If you cut yourself at the beach, remember to cleanse the wound thoroughly after you leave the salt water.

A clean cobweb is reported to sometimes be helpful in treating a cut in the woods. Cobwebs are reported to contain penicillin and other germ fighters.

Dental Problems

To help relieve the pain of a toothache, Thomas Gossel, Ph.D. at Ohio Northern University suggests massaging the back of your hand, in the dip between your thumb and index finger, with an ice cube. In U.S. Pharmacist magazine, Dr. Gossel reports that the ice cube treatment seems to relieve pain in the same way as acupuncture, but it doesn't matter whether you use the hand that is on the same side as the toothache or not.

Gum disease often occurs due to a weakening of the bones, known as osteoporosis. Preventing osteoporosis may also help prevent some cases of gum disease. (See: **Osteoporosis**)

Be sure to take out partial dentures at night to help maintain the good health of the gum tissues that support the partials. Keep partials and full dentures immaculately clean.

Replace your toothbrush every three months and only use a brush with soft bristles. Hard bristles may not damage your teeth, but they can damage your gums which are just as important to your dental health. Brush so that the bristles gently reach the gum line where the teeth and gums meet. This will help remove plaque build-up from the teeth under the gums and help to stimulate the gums. Brush at least twice daily, floss once each day and visit your dentist twice a year to maintain good dental health.

To prevent tooth decay in young children, follow these guidelines from the National Institute of Dental Research. If you must give your baby a bottle at bedtime, fill it only with water. Never allow your child to sleep with a bottle containing milk, formula, fruit juices or other sweet liquids. If your child needs a bottle for comfort, fill it with water or use a clean pacifier; NEVER dip the pacifier in any sugary liquid such as honey or syrup. After each feeding, clean your baby's teeth and gums with a damp washcloth or gauze pad. Start regular dental check-ups for your child by age 2 to 3 years.

After giving a child liquid medicine, be sure to have him rinse his mouth and brush his teeth. The sugar and stickiness of the liquid create an excellent environment for bacteria and tooth decay. Brushing the teeth will help eliminate the problem.

Depression

Pets can help people overcome loneliness and depression. Almost half of the psychologists, psychiatrists and family doctors who participated in a recent survey have prescribed "pet therapy" for emotional problems like depression and loneliness. Many doctors and therapists feel that pets provide love, support, an opportunity for exercise and a reason for living. By owning, loving and caring for a pet, people are reassured that they are needed. A renewed sense of self-worth and responsibility is established by having a pet. Many health professionals are now recommending the loving companionship and responsibility that a pet provides.

Vigorous exercise for a few minutes each day stimulates the brain and helps combat depression. A recent study found that in two groups of depressed patients, the patients who were encouraged to run everyday improved as much as the patients who received psychotherapy for their depression. Exercise seems to be most helpful for people suffering from depression associated with anxiety over a recent event. For people with anxiety because of a recent event, exercise may be as effective as prescription tranquilizers in calming nerves and tension or relieving the "jitters". Exercise may not be the complete cure for depression, but it is a healthy way to help deal with the problem.

People who are prone to depression and live in the northern United States should carefully plan for the winter months. With shorter days, longer periods of darkness and cold weather, many people suffer deep depressions in the winter. Suicides are more common in the winter in clinically depressed patients, according to studies by the National Institute of Mental Health. Making plans for special activities in the winter, establishing a strong social network of people whom you can contact even if you can't leave the house, growing houseplants and using plenty of bright, artificial lights in your environment can help fight off the winter blues.

Diabetes

A high-fiber diet during your lifetime may reduce your chances of getting diabetes later in life (known as maturity-onset diabetes). However, some cases of diabetes aren't caused by diet or obesity. In juvenile diabetes, there is a lack of insulin, possibly caused by a viral attack on the insulin-producing cells.

As you get older, your hormone levels naturally drop off. So obesity and unnatural eating habits put too much strain on your pancreas and you may become prone to maturity-onset diabetes. Diets which aren't low in fat or high in fiber make it difficult for insulin to bind to receptor sites. However, if you already have diabetes, be sure to check with your doctor before you go on a high-fiber, low-fat diet. Your doctor may have you on medication, and any change in your diet can upset the carefully balanced carbohydrate requirements that have been established for you.

Studies have shown that the mineral chromium can even out swings in blood sugar levels in people who have a tendency toward low blood sugar (hypoglycemia) or high blood sugar (hyperglycemia). Chromium supplements may aid in the treatment of maturity-onset diabetes and problems which are associated with diabetes, such as a tendency towards infections, hearing and circulatory problems. Adults need between 50 - 200 mcg. of chromium per day.

People with diabetes mellitus (sugar diabetes) who are taking insulin should consult their physicians before taking thiamine (Vitamin B1) supplements because large doses of thiamine may inactivate insulin.

Research has shown that people with diabetes may need extra vitamin C. However, diabetics may not be able to transport vitamin C into their cells. This may contribute to the blood vessel damage that diabetics experience.

Diabetics taking oral drugs to lower their blood sugar levels should not take vitamin C without the supervision of their physician, because vitamin C may block the action of these drugs.

Studies by Kurt A. Oster, M.D. and others indicate that large doses of folic acid may be helpful in the treatment and prevention of diabetes. Larger, controlled studies are necessary to confirm these small studies and reports of clinical experience.

People with diabetes are unusually prone to zinc deficiency, because diabetes lowers the blood levels of zinc. Adults need 15 mg. of zinc daily.

Supplementation of the mineral manganese has been reported to cause improvement in some cases of diabetes. The Recommended Daily Dietary Allowance (RDA) of manganese for adults is 2.5 - 5.0 mg. It is deficient in many diets.

New scientific reports claim that garlic may help in the fight against diabetes.

Aerobic exercise may help in managing diabetes. Dr. Daniel Delio in Brooklyn, New York says that diabetics should walk, swim, cycle, jog or run for the best exercise. Diabetics, especially those on insulin, should check with their doctor before starting an aerobic exercise program. To maintain good blood sugar levels, diabetics should exercise about one hour after eating and should drink plenty of fluids to avoid dehydration.

Diabetics often have problems with circulation, so daily attention should be given to the feet. Keep feet clean and dry; toenails should be clipped straight across; corns and calluses should be examined by a doctor or podiatrist. Care should be taken to buy shoes that fit well, are comfortable and are made of leather, not plastic or vinyl.

Diaper Rash

Diaper rash is a common occurrence that can easily be avoided or treated to cause minimal discomfort for the mother and the baby. If diaper rash is present, avoid using creams or petroleum jelly unless they are especially medicated for treating diaper rash, because they may seal the skin and prevent healing.

Since keeping the bottom dry is the most important step in avoiding diaper rash, change diapers frequently. Allow the baby to spend some time every day with a bare bottom by placing him on a dry diaper or a plastic sheet. Avoid using plastic pants or disposable diapers that have tight plastic linings. Use ultra-absorbent disposable diapers that don't form a tight seal at the legs. When using cloth diapers, wash them in mild detergent, since harsh detergents may cause irritation. Cornstarch powder can be used to help keep the baby's bottom dry. Be sure to sprinkle the powder in your hand and then use on the baby, because inhaling the dust can cause irritation to a baby's lungs.

Diarrhea

Diarrhea can be a bothersome reaction to stress, spicy foods or the body's attempting to rid itself of a virus. However, severe diarrhea can cause death by dehydration. It should be treated by intravenous fluid replacement in a hospital.

Mild diarrhea in children sometimes may be caused by allergies to juice. It seems that some children's digestive systems simply cannot tolerate apple, pear, or grape juice because they are high in carbohydrates.

Rice water, sweetened with corn syrup or sugar (1 teaspoon per 4 fluid ounces) is recommended for treating mild diarrhea in babies, according to Dr. James E. Strain at the University of Colorado. The water used to boil rice is acceptable for MILD diarrhea, because it helps replace the fluids and minerals which are lost. Plus, after fighting off the diarrhea, the bowel cannot properly digest lactose, the sugar in milk, so rice water is a better fluid for the child.

When treating diarrhea or an upset stomach with clear liquids, the American Journal of Diseases of Children suggests that the temperature of the liquid is just as important as the type of liquid. Cold liquids tend to stimulate the intestines and make diarrhea worse. Drinks that are room temperature or slightly warm are the best for diarrhea or stomach indigestion, says the Journal.

Honey and vinegar have long been recommended as a natural cure for diarrhea. However, the World Health Organization (WHO) suggests its own natural remedy that has a better balance of nutrients: combine 8 ounces of orange juice, a pinch of table salt and 1/2 teaspoon of honey or corn syrup; in a second glass, mix 8 ounces of distilled water and 1/4 teaspoon of baking soda. Alternate drinking sips from each glass.

Some diarrhea, unexplained gas and bloating is caused by the artificial sweetener sorbitol. "Excess consumption of sorbitol may have a laxative effect", according to the Food and Drug Administration (FDA). Sorbitol is found in many kinds of food products, including ice cream, gum, carbonated drinks, jelly and baked goods. It is also found naturally in some fruits, like prunes. If you consume a lot of sorbitol-containing products and are suffering from diarrhea or unexplained gas, try reading labels for listed ingredients and eliminating sorbitol from your diet.

To treat traveler's diarrhea, the Mayo Clinic recommends using a clear, liquid diet. Consume only weak tea, Seven-Up®, fruit juices (that are not made from concentrate), Jello® and soup broth.

During the day, you should drink some of this special Mayo Clinic preparation: 1/2 teaspoon table salt; 1/2 teaspoon baking soda; and 4 tablespoons of table sugar in 1 liter of carbonated water. (You can use plain water that has been boiled for 15 minutes if carbonated water is not available). As the diarrhea begins to improve, you can supplement the clear diet with semisolid and then solid foods.

To avoid getting "traveler's diarrhea" when on a trip, do not eat any fresh salads, fruits or vegetables unless you peel them yourself. Do not drink unpasteurized milk or other dairy products and never eat anything purchased from a street vendor. Avoid ordinary water, including ice in your drinks. Bottled water or water you have boiled is acceptable and should be used even for brushing your teeth. Eat only meat, poultry, fish, vegetables and eggs that have been thoroughly cooked in sanitary conditions.

Dizziness

Dizziness may be a sign of a serious illness, like heart problems or strokes, but many times dizziness is just a side effect of aspirin or another drug. Since aspirin is so commonly used, we sometimes forget that it is a drug and can cause serious side effects.

Dizziness can lead to dangerous falls or accidents

while driving.

Frequent dizzy spells should be reported to your doctor as soon as possible. If you are taking a lot of aspirin or any other drugs, be sure to tell the doctor all the medications you are taking, because the drugs may be the reason for the dizziness. (Geriatrics 41: 7, 31)

Dry Mouth

Thirst and dryness of the mouth can be caused by an overdose of calcium or vitamin D, or by a deficiency of potassium. A severe deficiency of sodium chloride (salt) can also cause dehydration.

Severe dry mouth may be a symptom of a serious disease or a side effect of a drug. There are many drugs that can cause dry mouth, including these commonly prescribed medications: Aldactone®, Aldomet®, Artane®, Benadryl®, Bentyl®, Catapres®, Cogentin®, Combid®, Dimetapp®, Donnatal®, Ditropan®, Elavil®, Flexeril®, Hydro-DIURIL®, Lasix®, Lomotil®, Mellaril®, Minipress®, nitroglycerin taken in pill form, Ornade®, Symmetrel®, Tenuate®, Triavil®, Valium® and many antihistamines.

Saliva helps to break down food particles, cleanse the teeth, prevent tooth decay and stimulate the taste buds, according to the National Institute of Dental Research. Therefore, it is important to treat a dry mouth.

People suffering from dry mouth should avoid cigarettes, alcohol and spicy, salty or highly acidic foods. Over-the-counter artificial salivas, Xero-Lube® and Moi-Stir®, can be used to help relieve dry mouth problems.

Ear Noises

Ringing in the ears or tinnitus (the medical term) is a serious problem for millions of Americans. In most cases, the cause is unknown and incurable. Some cases can be helped by avoiding alcohol, nicotine, marijuana, caffeine, aspirin products, prescription tranquilizers, oral contraceptives, quinine, overdoses of vitamin D or overexposure to the sun. Be sure to avoid exposure to loud noises like airplane motors, construction equipment, lawn mowers, loud music and gunshots. However, even these remedies don't work for everyone.

With daily zinc supplements, Dr. George Shambaugh, Jr., has reduced the problem of ear noises in over twenty patients at Northwestern University in Illinois. Dr. Shambaugh gives six hundred milligrams of zinc sulfate orally each day to reduce tinnitus. Because of possible side effects, such large doses should only be taken under a doctor's advice.

Some reports claim that a deficiency of the mineral, manganese, can cause ringing in the ears.

Manganese is naturally found in whole-grain products, fruits (especially bananas), eggs, vegetables (especially legumes), liver and other organ meats. A deficiency of the vitamin, choline, has been reported to cause noises in the ears. Choline forms part of the nervous system transmitter acetylcholine and is naturally found in lecithin, soybeans, eggs, fish, liver, wheat germ, green vegetables, peanuts, brewer's yeast, and sunflower seeds.

Masking the sound is often the best way to cope with minor ear noises. In ordinary circumstances, ear sounds are often not heard. In some cases, it's only when the room gets quiet that the ear noises become unbearable. The constant sound of a TV, radio, fan, air conditioner or heater may help "cover up" the sound of the ear noises. At night, when trying to fall asleep, try setting your clock radio on the sleep setting, so the noise of the radio will mask the sounds in your ears. Or, try setting the radio between stations. Even the sound of the static may help drown out annoying ear noises.

Some people find that the ear noises bother them only when they are extremely tired or under pressure. Try getting plenty of rest and avoid stress to see if that eliminates or lowers the intensity of your ear noises.

In some rare cases, a loose hair in the ear canal can cause loud noises. Dr. George Goldman of Massachusetts Institute of Technology (MIT) has treated several patients complaining of ear noises who have had an ear hair floating close to the ear drum. When the loose hair vibrates, it causes unusually loud noises that sound like "distant thunder". When the hair is removed, by rinsing the ear with water or by forceps, the sounds disappear. If you have had a haircut just prior to experiencing ear noises, a loose hair may have caused the problem.

Ear Problems

Ear problems should be carefully handled, since the ear canal is so fragile and so important. Itching in the ear is usually caused by a lack of ear wax which creates a dry ear canal, says Dr. Jeffrey C. Reynolds of Hays, Kansas. Without the ear wax, the ear becomes dry, red and itchy and will be sensitive to wind blowing in the ear or cold air. To avoid itchy ears, occasionally applying a small amount of baby oil, petroleum jelly, or glycerine with your little finger may help relieve dryness. DO NOT use cotton-tipped applicators. To prevent dryness and itching, make sure that soap or shampoo does not get in the ear canals, or rinse the ears thoroughly after exposure to soapy water. Tilt your head from side to side to get rid of any soap. If you still suspect that soap is left in the ear canal, rinse the ear with a dilute mixture of salt water.

Swimmer's ear is a common ear infection caused by small organisms in the ear canal. Once swimmer's ear occurs, the doctor should be consulted for antibiotics. However, to prevent swimmer's ear, avoid swimming in ponds or slow moving bodies of water. Completely dry your ears after swimming or diving by shaking your head and fanning your ears. If necessary, use a hair dryer to help dry your ears. DON'T use a cotton-tipped applicator. After swimming, one doctor suggests applying two drops of a homemade solution into each ear. Use two tablespoons of boiled water and thirty drops of white vinegar. Wait for the solution to cool before putting it in the ears.

Removing bugs from ears can be a tricky and dangerous project. Do not spray or use a bug killer in the ear, because it could damage the ear drum. The <u>Emergency Medical</u> journal (13-6: 122) recommends taking the person with a live bug in their ear into a completely dark room, like a closet. Shine a flashlight into the ear. The flashlight will attract the bug which will then crawl right out of the ear. Dead bugs must be floated out or taken out with a syringe by a doctor.

Edema: See **Fluid Retention**

Eye Problems

Itching, burning eyes, night blindness or loss of vision in near darkness are some of the early symptoms of vitamin A deficiency. Vitamin A can naturally be obtained in liver, cod liver oil, eggs, whole milk products, broccoli, spinach, and other green leafy vegetable. Carotene, which a healthy body can convert into vitamin A, is found in yellow fruits and vegetables, like carrots.

Chronic red eyes may be caused by a lack of tears. Sometimes, dry eyes are caused by changes in the hormonal balance in a woman, an environment that is too dry or windy or overexposure to the sun. Artificial tears, available over-the-counter, may help. Sleeping with a bedroom humidifier, protecting the eyes with wrap around sunglasses and avoiding exposure to wind, sun or dirty air may help reduce dryness.

Long hours in front of a video display terminal (VDT) screen can cause eye strain, fatigue and neck problems, according to Robert C. Yeager, contributor to the Medical and Health Annual published by Encyclopaedia Britannica, Inc. If you are using a VDT, Yeager recommends using good support lighting, a one-color, high contrast, low-glare screen, and taking breaks at least every two hours. Doing eye exercises and using a good supportive chair may also help reduce discomfort caused by VDT use.

Protecting our eyes is important to keep our eyesight throughout our lives. Here are several easy steps to prevention recommended by The National Society to Prevent Blindness.

To avoid loss of your eyesight, have frequent eye check-ups if you have high blood pressure, diabetes or a history of vision problems. Pain in the eyes, excessive discharge from the eyes, loss of vision, dry eyes, double vision, swelling or redness of the eye or eyelid are possible warning signs of vision problems and should be checked immediately by an eye doctor. Even if you do not experience any loss of vision, you should have a regular eye exam by an ophthamologist at least once every two years, so that possible problems can be detected early.

Wear sunglasses that transmit no more than 30 percent of light to the eyes. Ultraviolet rays can damage the eyes and increase your chances of developing cataracts or eye cancer. According to the New England Journal of Medicine (13, 313), a deadly cancer of the eye, called intraocular malignant melanoma, is most likely to occur in people who have spent a lot of time outdoors, sunbathers or people who use sun lamps. You can lower your risk by wearing protective sunglasses, hats, or visors while in the sun. Sitting under an umbrella at the beach may protect you from direct sunlight, but the dangerous rays bounce off the sand and back under the umbrella. Even under an umbrella, you should still protect your eyes and wear a sunscreen to protect your skin. Being on sand, snow or a large body of water will increase your exposure to the rays if you are not protected.

Never look directly into the sun. Many people irreversibly damage their eyes by looking at the sun. Just because it may not be painful does not mean that staring into the sun is not harmful.

Don't share any items that touch your eyes with someone else. Eye make-up, towels or eye make-up applicators should never be used by more than one person. Throw away old eye make-up since it can easily become contaminated.

Never wet eye make-up or contact lenses with your saliva. Saliva from your mouth carries many kinds of bacteria and can cause dangerous eye infections.

Use adequate lighting for all demanding visual tasks like reading, watching TV, cooking and handicrafts. Use regular lightbulbs (incandescent light) instead of tubular overhead lights (fluorescent light). Incandescent light is easier on the eyes. Try to avoid straining the eyes.

Use protective safety-glasses when working around industrial equipment or power tools, bicycling, playing racquet sports or swimming.

Don't rub your eye if you get a speck in it. "Lift the upper eyelid outward and down over the lower lid, and let the tears wash out the speck or particle", says the National Society To Prevent Blindness.

Fatigue
Adults, especially women before the menopause and the elderly, may suffer from fatigue caused by iron deficiency. Parents of children suffering from fatigue, tiredness or irritability should make sure that both the child and the mother have enough iron in their diets. Dr. Lawrence Wolfe, a Boston pediatrician, says many children between 6 to 18 months are iron-deficient and suffer from behavior problems. To ensure enough daily iron, young children and their mothers (if breast-feeding) should eat whole-grain products, liver, organ meats, eggs, fish, raisins, tomatoes, green vegetables, and cereals that are fortified with iron. If you are taking iron supplements, follow dosage directions; don't overdose on iron.

Getting a good night's sleep is important to avoid being tired or suffering from fatigue. Sleep on a comfortable bed, keep your room well-ventilated and at a comfortable temperature, and get between 8 - 10 hours of sleep each night, depending on your individual needs. Also see: **Insomnia**.

Quit smoking. Not only can smoking cause hardening of the arteries and lung cancer, it limits the amount of oxygen the blood can process. Since the blood cannot use the oxygen properly, smokers are more inclined to suffer from fatigue.

In some cases, fatigue can actually be helped by exercise. A brisk walk or swim before breakfast may really help overcome morning tiredness. The physical activity will help get the blood circulating and make more oxygen available to the body. The increased oxygen supply will help stimulate the whole body, including the brain. After exercise, be sure to eat breakfast.

Fatigue and tiredness may be caused by skipping or skimping on breakfast. According to a recent study, people who suffered from fatigue often skipped breakfast. They experienced less fatigue when they ate high protein breakfasts, including meat, fish, cheese (mozzarella, provolone or cottage), or egg whites with two tablespoons of brewer's yeast.

Some people discover their fatigue is reduced if they eat smaller, yet more frequent meals throughout the day. Eating small portions of food, perhaps six times a day, seems to keep the body's energy at a constant level.

Have your eyes examined. Improper glasses or contacts can put great strain on your eyes and zap your energy. An eye exam may discover a visual problem that has been causing your tiredness.

Lose weight. Think of how much strain carrying a 20 pound sack of potatoes would put on your body, then ask yourself if you are 20 pounds overweight. The extra pounds you carry put additional stress and strain on your heart, circulatory system and the whole body. The extra stress may drain the body's energy, resulting in tiredness. Proper nutrition and good eating habits will help you lose weight, fight fatigue and improve your overall health.

Change your routine. Any tedious routine, at home or at work, can cause tiredness and feelings of depression. Try doing something spontaneously and change your daily schedule if possible. This may help reduce tiredness, fatigue and depression.

Extreme fatigue, combined with an intolerance to cold, weight gain and achy muscles, may be caused by a thyroid gland problem. The thyroid gland produces a hormone called thyroxine, that is essential for all the body's metabolic processes. If the thyroid doesn't produce enough hormone, called hypothyroidism, your body's metabolism will start to slow down. Hypothyroidism is quite common and can easily be treated by prescription drugs. If you suspect this condition, visit your doctor as soon as possible.

Fever

Fever helps the body fight infections, so low fevers should not routinely be lowered. However, if your fever goes above 103°F or stays above 100°F for three days, you should see a doctor. Fever can be a sign of a serious illness that should be treated by a doctor. You should only try to lower a fever under your doctor's advice.

For adults, plain aspirin can be taken to reduce the fever. Do NOT use aspirin compounds that include caffeine, like Anacin® or Excedrin®, since caffeine increases body temperature.

However, children should be given acetaminophen. Do NOT give children aspirin. Children with a fever who are given aspirin may increase their risk of getting Reye's syndrome, a sometimes fatal disease that affects the liver and brain.

The person with a fever should be allowed to rest comfortably. Drinking plenty of liquids, at least two quarts of water and/or juice a day, is very important. With every degree the body temperature rises, the body loses a pint of fluid per day. Drinking liquids helps the body from becoming dehydrated as it is fighting off the fever and infection. Do NOT use any liquids that contain caffeine, like coffee, tea, or cola drinks, because caffeine increases body temperature.

If the person with the fever is complaining about the heat, a cool washcloth placed on his forehead may make him feel better. It doesn't really do much to reduce the fever, but a cold compress often makes the fever easier to tolerate.

Make sure that perspiration can evaporate from the feverish person's skin. Using cotton sleepwear, sheets and underwear is best. Do not force the feverish person to be covered under layers of heavy comforters and blankets. Heavy blankets will not allow sweat to evaporate, and the feverish person's temperature will not be able to correct itself.

Fever Blisters

Fever blisters affect over 70 percent of the population at one time or another. They are annoying blisters that are caused by a herpes simplex virus infection. They usually appear as clear, fluid-filled sacs on the lips, in the nostrils or in the mouth.

Avoiding acidic foods, like citrus juices and fruits, and high-fat foods, may help reduce the number of fever blisters or the length of time they are active, says Robert J. Peshek, D.D.S. in the Journal of Applied Nutrition. Dr. Peshek recommends eating plenty of alkaline foods, like vegetables, bananas and skim milk and taking vitamin B complex supplements. Avoiding stress, sunburn, emotional upset, colds or fever may also help keep fever blisters from breaking out. Dr. Peshek believes that so many things can affect the eruption of fever blisters that it is best to attack on all fronts, including nutrition, rest and stress reduction.

Several doctors and dentists have applied vitamin E directly onto fever blisters to help them heal faster and reduce the pain. Don E. Nead, D.D.S. of Redding, California applies vitamin E in oil, on a piece of gauze, directly to the fever blister for about 15 minutes.

In a recent study at Baylor University School of Medicine, lysine supplements cut the rate of fever blister eruption in half, after the supplements were taken for six months

A letter in one medical journal suggested placing an ice cube on a newly erupted fever blister, preferably for about 45 minutes. Some people who get fever blisters regularly use the ice cube treatment BEFORE the blisters erupt. (If you get these blisters very often, you can recognize their presence by a "hot spot" before they start showing.) The ice cube treatment may not stop the fever blister from showing, but it can shorten the length of time the blister is painfully active. Camphor and phenol lotions applied to newly erupted blisters can shrink the blisters and relieve pain.

Fibrocystic Breast Disease: See Breast Disease — Fibrocystic

Fluid Retention

Fluid retention is the excessive accumulation of fluid in the body tissues, medically referred to as edema or dropsy. Fluid retention can be the result of an inflammation or an illness, like congestive heart disease, so be sure to check with your doctor to see if medical treatment is necessary.

Some women suffer from a weight gain of up to five pounds of fluid, particularly just prior to menstruation. In women, an increase in estrogen levels (occurring during pregnancy, during the menstrual cycle and when taking oral contraceptives) increases the body's need for pyridoxine. Pyridoxine (vitamin B6) supplements may, therefore, help relieve or reduce the symptoms of pre-menstrual fluid retention, weight gain, pre-menstrual acne, depression and menopausal arthritis. Serious side effects have been reported after taking large doses of B6, more than 25 mg. per day. Potassium supplements are claimed to help reduce fluid retention, but be careful not to exceed the daily dose recommendations for potassium.

Prolonged deficiency of thiamine (vitamin B1) can lead to fluid retention and swelling in the hands and feet.

To help prevent excess fluid retention: exercise regularly; lose weight; avoid salt; rest your legs and feet at least twice a day by lying with your feet higher than your heart; wear support panty-hose when possible; and avoid eating black licorice or licorice extracts because they may contribute to salt and fluid retention. About 90% of the licorice imported into the United States is used in chewing tobacco. This is another reason people should avoid all forms of tobacco use.

Food Allergies

Food allergies can cause symptoms like headache, upset stomach, diarrhea, unwell feelings, rapid heartbeat, hives, or shock. Check with your doctor and get his okay for self-treatment. Many migraine headache sufferers have found that they may be allergic to certain foods that seem to trigger severe headaches. A recent test involving children revealed that migraine headaches disappeared in 85% of the children when they went on a diet without many of the foods which commonly cause allergies, according to Postgraduate Medicine (75-4, 221). After withdrawal, the foods were reintroduced one by one, over a long period of time, so the allergic reactions would be noticed and associated with the offending foods. The foods and additives that caused the headaches, in order of the most offending foods, are: cow's milk, egg, chocolate, orange, wheat, benzoic acid (a preservative), cheese, tomatoes, yellow-dye # 5, rye, fish, pork, beef, corn and soy. Other foods that are known to cause common allergies include: green peas and other legumes, peanuts, licorice, lima beans, shellfish and other seafood, fruits that have pits and berries. Please also see: **Headaches**.

To truly determine if a food allergy is present, the symptoms of the allergy must disappear when the food is removed from the diet and reappear when the food is reintroduced. Reintroducing a food is not recommended if the allergic reaction was serious or life-threatening.

Keeping a detailed journal of your diet and the symptoms you experience may be valuable in identifying your food allergies. Every food and drink must be carefully recorded, including the precise amount of food, how it was prepared and when it was eaten or drunk. Write down everything you eat and drink, including the various ingredients, spices, condiments, vitamins, prescription or over-the-counter drugs. Weigh yourself every morning. If you notice any weight loss or gain, weigh yourself twice daily. Be sure to write down any food or beverage cravings you experience during the time you are keeping the journal. Describe the reactions, how long they lasted and at what time they occurred. Over a period of time, this journal will help you to notice trends in your reactions.

It is important to fast, or avoid all selected foods for five days before beginning a food allergy test. Dr. Marshall Mandell, a renowned clinical ecologist, recommends eating only one food per meal, and not eating that food again for at least 5 to 7 days. This will give the body enough time to completely rid itself of the food allergen. Then, a very noticeable reaction will take place when the offending food is eaten.

In some people, an allergic food reaction may cause an increase in pulse rate. Although this occurs only one-third of the time, it can be used with other techniques to help verify an allergy. The pulse test was first described by Arthur F. Coca, M.D. in The Pulse Test published by Lyle Stuart in 1967. After determining your normal pulse, check your pulse after eating suspect foods.

An elimination diet is especially helpful in spotting offending foods for people who may be allergic to several different foods. After you have kept a food and symptoms journal, you should have some suspicions about certain foods. Set up the elimination diet based on your journal findings. Don't eat food that you already know you are allergic to, just the foods that you are not sure of. Try to avoid processed foods because they make it difficult to determine whether the processing ingredients, or the food itself, is causing the allergy. While on a rotation diet, try preparing each food very simply — like baking or steaming, or eating fruits and vegetables raw. Remember, you want to avoid any cooking methods, spices, or outside factors that could alter the results of the diet.

As well as a method of determining food allergies, rotation diets are one way to avoid allergic food reactions. Many people can just rotate their foods every seven days and not suffer from allergic attacks. Most people with food allergies eat the same food several times during a short period of time and compound the problem. Rotation diets are often used if someone doesn't have time for testing and keeping a journal. Because the rotation diet helps eliminate overeating of foods, a person may feel better without ever discovering the actual allergy. However, if a severe allergy is present the rotation diet won't help; the food should simply be completely avoided.

Cutting down on food variety may help eliminate food allergies. Try just a few foods and eat a lot of them at meals, rather than mixing a lot of different food groups. Use fresh, unprocessed food as much as possible.

If you believe you are suffering from allergies, do not drink any alcohol. Alcohol may speed up an allergic reaction. Do not eat any suspect food on an empty stomach, because doing this may turn a mild reaction into a severe reaction. Be very careful with your diet during hay-fever season, because you may be more sensitive at that time. Be wary of any foods in the same family group of foods that may cause allergies.

Allergies may be caused by a food additive, packaging material, pesticide used when the food is grown, food color, flavoring, emulsifier, preservative, or stabilizer. Allergies can also be caused by natural flavorings like cinnamon, vanilla or peppermint.

Consider growing as much of your own food as possible or buy your food from local growers who don't use extensive insecticides and chemicals. Locally grown food helps to avoid the polishes and other additives that are often put on fresh fruits and vegetables at grocery stores.

If you are allergic to chemicals in your water, try bottled water. Buy bottled water in glass containers, since chemicals can seep into water from plastic containers. Invest in a home water filter, if possible.

Watch the packaging you are buying and storing your food in. Try to avoid using plastic wrap and plastic containers. Use glass jars for storing. Buy food in bulk to avoid unnecessary packaging.

Children who are born to parents with allergies often have allergies, too. To reduce allergies in newborns, doctors recommend: (1) the mother should avoid all possibly allergic foods for the last three months of pregnancy and while breast-feeding, (2) breast-feed for the first year (or use a hypoallergenic formula if necessary), (3) when solid foods are introduced, use a rotation plan.

Introduce one food at a time and rotate it with just a few other foods, and watch for any unusual reactions to the new foods. Don't introduce different foods all at once.

Foot Odors

Fighting smelly feet can be quite simple if you follow these suggestions. Go barefoot or wear open sandals without socks as much as possible, so the air will allow the feet to breathe. When wearing socks, use lightweight cotton socks, because better air-flow to the feet allows the sweat to evaporate. Wash the feet thoroughly and often, being sure to dry them completely. Applying plain talcum powder or baking soda between the toes after drying may be helpful. Try never to wear the same pair of shoes two days in a row. Alternating shoes will give them more time to dry out and prevent the build-up of foot odors. Buy and wear leather shoes, rather than plastic or synthetic shoes, because leather allows the shoes to breathe.

Freckles: See **Skin Problems**

Frostbite

Skin that is exposed to cold air for too long a time

or is exposed to low temperatures combined with fierce winds may become frostbitten. Frostbite usually occurs on the hands, nose, face, ears, toes and feet. These areas on the body's outer extremities are more exposed to the cold, and, thus, are more susceptible to frostbite.

In the first stages of frostbite, the affected areas may turn white or yellow, and loss of feeling, burning, or itching is experienced. However, since there may be no discomfort, frostbite can go unnoticed.

The best treatment is to gently warm the area. A mitten placed against frostbite on the face can help. The frostbitten person should return inside, preferably to a warm, but not hot, environment. If you notice frostbite, but cannot return to a shelter, try warming your frostbitten parts with the warmth of other body parts. If your hand has become frostbitten, hold it underneath your armpit. If your toes are affected, try holding your hands against them. Wrap the frostbitten area in a warm blanket, if possible.

DO NOT rub frostbitten skin either with your hands or with snow. Warm, gentle heat is the best way to thaw the frozen skin. If the frostbitten skin is exposed to heat that is too hot, it may be damaged, since the numbed skin cannot feel the heat. Drink lots of hot liquids. Avoid smoking, because it constricts blood vessels, which need to stay open to warm the frostbite.

To prevent frostbite, dress warmly and in layers to help allow your body to breathe while you are outdoors in cold weather. Protect your head. Almost 50% of your body's heat loss is through your head, so be sure to wear a warm hat and earmuffs. Scarves can help protect your neck and face. Buy and wear gloves or mittens that are comfortable and provide good insulation.

Gallstones

Dr. Heaton of England's Bristol University recommends a low-calorie, low-fat, high-fiber diet with special emphasis upon a restricted intake of refined carbohydrates (sugar) to prevent gallstones. The British Medical Journal reports that vegetarians are less likely to suffer from gallstones than non-vegetarians. A natural remedy is two weeks on a balanced diet, followed by three days on fruit juice, then treatment of half a pint of olive oil and half a pint of lemon juice once a day, with only water to drink the rest of the time. The oil may help the gallstones pass naturally.

We can't confirm how safe or successful this treatment might be or if there are side effects, so don't try it unless your doctor wants you to.

Lecithin, a substance extracted from egg yolks, soybeans and other high-fat foods, is thought to be important in keeping liver cell membranes healthy and perhaps reducing the chance of getting gallstones, according to Tim Watkins of the City University of New York. The manufacturer of Lipton® soup is reported to be hoping to capitalize on this study by selling a new "healthy" soup containing 80% pure lecithin.

According to researchers at Flinders Medical Center in Australia, one ounce of alcohol per day reduced the risk of developing gallstones. Studies show that high amounts of alcohol, sugar and fat increase the risk of getting gallstones, but this recent research showed that just a small amount of alcohol each day actually decreased the risk factor.

Gas

Beans, milk and milk products, broccoli, brussel sprouts, carbonated drinks, melons, apples and wheat-flour products all cause gas in some people. Try eliminating these foods, one by one, to see if you can determine which ones give you problems. Then, permanently eliminate the foods that give you problems.

Great stress can also cause gas problems. Try to reduce the stressful factors in your lifestyle.

Also see: **Stress**

Also see: **Indigestion**

Hair Problems

Dry and brittle hair may be caused by a deficiency of vitamin A, vitamin C or iodine.

Defects in the pigmentation and structure of the hair may be caused by a deficiency of the mineral copper. Copper helps in the formation of hair, bone and skin.

To keep your hair soft and shiny, protect it from the ultraviolet rays of the sun by wearing a scarf or hat. Wash it with a shampoo that will help your type of hair, dry, oily or normal. Avoid or limit the use of blow drying, hot curlers and curling irons, because they damage the hair. Allow your hair to dry naturally or towel dry it, but never rub your hair, just pat it dry. Always rinse your hair after exposure to chlorine in a swimming pool or salt in sea water. Never color your hair and get a permanent at the same time. Give your hair time to adjust between each major process.

Wash your hair with a shampoo and apply a separate conditioner, rather than a shampoo with an added conditioner. Leave the conditioner on for at least five minutes, preferably with your hair wrapped in a warm towel. Change shampoo and conditioner for a two week period every six weeks. This may help stop the detergents in one particular kind of shampoo from building up and damaging your hair. If you have two brands of shampoo that you like, rotate them to help avoid build-up problems.

Hangovers

Hangovers usually occur the morning after consuming too much alcohol the evening before. Headaches, body aches, upset stomach and tiredness are all symptoms of a hangover. The Food and Drug Administration (FDA) recommends: caffeine for the tiredness, aspirin for the headaches, and an antacid for the upset stomach. Sleeping and avoiding loud music or noise is also recommended.

The best remedy is prevention: avoid overconsumption of alcoholic beverages, especially whiskey which contains chemicals which cause bad hangovers.

Headaches

People who suffer from migraine headaches should try these simple suggestions from the Emergency Medicine journal (16-14: 69). Reduce the amount of caffeine you consume daily. Avoid foods that contain TYRAMINE like chicken livers or old cheese. Avoid or limit sodium glutamate, a preservative in processed foods, and sodium nitrate, which is found in cured meats like ham and hot dogs. Eat regular meals at the same time each day to avoid swings in blood sugar levels. Avoid or limit carbohydrates, especially sugars, and avoid oral contraceptives or ESTROGEN.

Other common causes of headaches include: sudden withdrawal from caffeine, bright, fluorescent, or pulsating lights, odors from perfume, after-shave, cologne, soap or detergent. Eating ice cream or frozen treats can cause headaches after the cold dessert hits the roof of the mouth. An overdose of salt, like you can get after eating a bowl of salted nuts or potato chips, bright sunlight, and alcohol (especially red wine) can also be culprits.

Food allergies cause symptoms like headache, upset stomach, diarrhea, unwell feelings, rapid heartbeat, hives, or shock. First, check with your doctor and get his okay for self-treatment. Many migraine headache sufferers have found that they may be allergic to certain foods that seem to trigger severe headaches. A recent test involving children discovered that the headaches disappeared in 85% of the children when on a diet without many of the foods which commonly cause allergies, according to Postgraduate Medicine (75-4, 221). After withdrawal, the foods were reintroduced one by one, over a long period of time, so the allergic reactions would be noticed and associated with the offending foods. The foods and additives that caused the headaches, in order of the most offending foods, are: cow's milk, egg, chocolate, orange, wheat, benzoic acid (a preservative), cheese, tomatoes, yellow-dye # 5, rye, fish, pork, beef, corn and soy. Other foods that are known to cause common allergies include: green peas and other legumes, peanuts, licorice, lima beans, shellfish and other seafood, fruits that have pits and berries. Also see: **Food Allergies**.

Researchers at National Hospital for Nervous Diseases in London have discovered that headaches can be triggered by foods with sodium cromoglycate (chromalyn), a protective chemical added to milk, wheat and eggs. The same people did not suffer from headaches when they received the same foods without the chromalyn additive. The researchers believe that many migraines may be caused by chemical additives in our food, rather than the food itself.

Kenneth Weaver, M.D. at East Tennessee State University believes that magnesium helps reduce and prevent migraines. Based on his findings with pregnant women, 100 milligrams per day is the optimal amount of magnesium needed to reduce headaches.

Fifteen one-gram fish oil capsules taken daily, brought dramatic relief to severe migraine headache sufferers in a study at the University of Cincinnati Medical Center. Researcher Robert Hitzmann, Ph.D., who worked on the study, believes that the fish oil contains a substance, omega-3 fatty acids, that inhibits the body's production of prostaglandins. Prostaglandin secretion is thought to play a role in causing severe migraine headaches. Another, smaller, study at the State University of New York at Stony Brook also reported that over 50% of people with migraines improved with fish oil treatment. Nutritionists, however, are recommending incorporating more fish into the regular diet, by eating fish at least twice a week, rather than taking capsule supplements. Salmon, mackerel, tuna, sardines, crab, shrimp, lobster and other shellfish are all high in beneficial omega-3 fatty acids if they aren't canned. Canning destroys most of the omega-3 fatty acids.

Biofeedback, a method of learning to relax bodily functions, has been used at Louisiana State University to lower the number of migraine headaches children suffer. According to the <u>Journal</u> <u>of</u> <u>Consulting</u> <u>and</u> <u>Clinical</u> <u>Psychology</u> (12, 84, 968) children between 7 and 16 years were trained in skin temperature biofeedback. The children learned how to warm their hands by directing their blood flow to their extremities. They practiced this technique twice a day and recorded the timing and severity of their headaches. This biofeedback technique also helps to regulate blood flow in the head. This helps reduce headaches, because some migraines are caused by a sudden change in the flow of blood in the head. All the children who received the biofeedback training experienced fewer and less severe headaches. Drs. Elise Labbe and Donald Williamson, who conducted the studies in Baton Rouge, are very excited about the findings, since drug-free treatment in children is so important.

If you suffer from headaches in the early morning, check to see if you are getting enough oxygen while you sleep. Make sure your room is ventilated. Don't sleep with your face in the pillow so you have enough oxygen to breathe while you sleep. You may also want to grow some broad-leaved house plants in your bedroom. They will add a little oxygen and moisture to the air.

Eating breakfast, or drinking a glass of orange juice in the morning will help prevent headaches by maintaining your body's blood sugar level. If you don't eat breakfast, your blood sugar level can drop and cause headaches, according to Dr. Edward Pinchney of Beverly Hills, California.

Severe headaches during sex may occur due to muscle or blood vessel contractions or the internal release of spinal fluid into the head during intercourse, according to Dr. Donald Johns in Archives of Neurology. Pain relievers or muscle relaxants may help eliminate this type of headache.

Folk medicine has been put to the test by doctors at the City of London Migraine Clinic, where they tested leaves from the feverfew plant to treat migraine headaches. Common feverfew is a plant in the chrysanthemum family. In patients who had used feverfew leaves as a remedy for their migraines, a three-fold increase in headaches and nausea was noticed when the patients received a placebo instead of the herb. (The capsules containing the herb or the placebo were identical and neither the researchers nor the patients knew when they were receiving what.) Many people prone to headaches eat four feverfew leaves a day to prevent headaches, while other people experience side effects and find they cannot tolerate the plant. Some health food stores in Britain and the U.S. are starting to carry feverfew supplements.

Some simple, drug-free remedies have also been successful for many people. Rest in a dark room with feet slightly elevated. Put ice compresses on the forehead or the back of the neck. Sit in the shower, alternating hot then cold water over the head and upper back.

Also see: **Temporomandibular Joint (TMJ) Dysfunctions.**

Heart Attacks

There are many risk factors which may affect the likelihood of your having a heart attack. These factors include: high blood pressure, a history of heart disease or heart attacks in your family, smoking, eating foods that are high in fat or cholesterol, being overweight, taking birth control pills, and taking over-the-counter diet pills containing phenylpropanolamine (PPA).

Regular supplements of the "heart protecting" vitamins C and E and the mineral selenium may not prevent a heart attack, but they may help to keep the heart living through the trauma of a heart attack, according to Joe McCord at the University of South Alabama College of Medicine. Since the worst damage to the heart often occurs immediately after the heart attack, McCord claims that if the body has an adequate supply of vitamins C and E and selenium, the heart muscle will have a better chance to survive.

Lifestyles and stress can affect each person's chances for survival following a heart attack. According to research published in The New England Journal of Medicine (311:552) loneliness and high levels of stress decrease the chances for survival in a person recovering from a heart attack. People who were not able to communicate effectively with their doctors or other medical staff or were not able to discuss things with family or close friends, or didn't participate in many social events had a lower survival rate than people who had a supportive and close family. Patients who participated in social and church activities and felt that they could talk to their doctors about their problems experienced quicker recoveries. Stress factors, such as not being satisfied with work, serious family problems or being connected with violent events, also decrease a patient's chances for survival after a heart attack. Therefore, to increase your chances for survival after a heart attack, avoid stressful situations, remain or become socially active, and draw close to your family, friends and church.

If you live in a climate with a severe winter, avoid unnecessary stress on your heart and circulation system. Dress properly and don't overexpose yourself to cold weather. Avoid physical exertion, especially shoveling snow, in the cold outdoors. Shoveling snow places great stress on the arms, muscles in the upper body, and the cardiovascular system. Each year, many people die of heart attacks that occur while shoveling snow. Buying a snowblower or hiring a young person to shovel the walks and driveway may be a good investment to prevent a heart attack.

Pets may be helpful in increasing your chances of survival after a heart attack. According to one study of 92 patients, 11 of the 29 people without pets died within a year of their hospitalization. However, only 3 of the 59 people who had pets died. With many other variables in the study like exercise, proper nutrition and diet, the study does not prove that pets alone improve survival rates. However, many doctors and therapists feel that pets provide love, support, an opportunity for exercise and a reason for living. Even though heart-attack patients have to rely on others for care, by having a pet they are reassured that something needs to depend on them. A renewed sense of self-worth and responsibility is established by having a pet. Pets also help people fight loneliness and depression which can be devastating after a heart-attack.

Heartburn: See **Indigestion**

Heart Pain: See **Angina Pectoris**

Heat Rash
Heat rash is small red bumps that appear on the skin after exposure to too much heat. When the skin's pores are blocked or don't produce enough sweat to cool off the body, heat rash can occur. To treat heat rash, first, get out of the heat. Drink lots of cool or cold liquids and bathe in cool water. Avoid using any lotion or cream, because lotion can block the pores and keep heat from being released through the skin. Aloe vera juice, directly from a plant, may be helpful, but don't use a cream or lotion even if it contains some aloe vera.

Hemorrhoids

Most hemorrhoids are caused by a diet lacking in fiber. Because of the lack of fiber, the stool matter is dry and hard, and bowel movements put a great strain on the rectal area. The best way to prevent hemorrhoids is to eat a diet high in bran, whole grain products, nuts, and fresh vegetables.

Hemorrhoids often afflict pregnant women, because of extra pressure, as well as people with jobs that require many hours of sitting. These people should be particularly careful to eat a high-fiber diet, get plenty of exercise, including walking for at least 10 minutes every two hours, and exercising the rectal muscles by squeezing and releasing them several times daily.

If you develop hemorrhoids after you have changed your eating habits to include more fiber, you may need to try these methods while you are waiting for the hemorrhoids to subside: soak in a tub of hot water, (or 1/4 cup witch hazel in a basin of warm water) three or four times a day; lie on your side or your stomach rather than sitting; keep your rectal area very clean; try applying a bag of ice to relieve swelling in the inflamed area; use moistened toilet paper to avoid aggravating the area; do not scratch hemorrhoids, because it will only cause further irritation.

Developing good toilet habits is also important to prevent hemorrhoids from occurring. Always go to the restroom when you need to go. If you put off going, your body will eventually lose its natural mechanism which tells you when to have a bowel movement. Never sit and strain to have a bowel movement — if you are eating properly, with enough fiber in your diet, bowel movements should be quick and natural. You should usually be able to have a bowel movement with little effort on your part. Just relax and let your body work on its own. Never use commercial laxatives or enemas — natural laxatives like prunes, raisins, other dried fruit and bran should be part of your regular diet. Commercial laxatives destroy the body's own ability to eliminate waste properly. If you start taking them, you may be caught in a vicious circle where you have to rely on them.

Hiccups

Hiccups can be caused by many things, including eating too quickly, eating too much, drinking too much alcohol, stress, or eating food that is too hot or too cold. Here are some suggestions for curing hiccups. These are "doctor" recommended methods to try in addition to the traditional methods of holding your breath, or blowing into a paper bag.

First, try stretching the diaphragm. The diaphragm is the muscle between your stomach and lungs. Hold your hands together behind your head and slowly lean backwards. Then take a deep breath while pulling your elbows back. You should feel as if you are releasing your stomach muscles. Or try lying down on a bed or sofa with your head and shoulders over the edge, then clasp your hands behind your head and stretch.

Another suggestion is to use a cotton-tipped swab to "tickle" or "massage" the back of the throat. Touch the upper back part of the throat, right where the roof of your mouth changes from bone to soft pink flesh. Try massaging the roof of your mouth for one or two minutes, and the hiccups should end. (U.S. Pharmacist 8-6: 33).

Other folk remedies, which seem to work by stimulating the nervous system, are: place chips of ice in your mouth; swallow a teaspoonful of dry granulated sugar or a little hard bread; hold your tongue and gently pull it forward; swallow water from the "wrong side" of a glass; drink water through a paper towel over a glass; drink sips of honey or vinegar; breathe pepper until you start sneezing; or suck on a lemon wedge.

Impotence
Impotence can be caused by a variety of psychological and physical reasons. Doctors have recently discovered that "hardening of the arteries", which is a major factor in heart disease, heart attacks and

strokes, can also lead to impotence. Studies in Paris, France, reported in the medical journal, <u>The Lancet</u>, showed that men who have cardiovascular disease risk factors, like diabetes or high blood pressure, those who smoke or have high concentrations of blood fats (lipids) are at increased risk for suffering from impotence. A man's ability to achieve an erection is based on a good blood supply to the penis, so hardening of the arteries can cause impotence. Doctors recommend that men with impotence problems should follow the same lifestyle changes as those recommended for people with cardiovascular problems: reduce the amount of cholesterol and fats in the diet, quit smoking and maintain a regular exercise program. Many cases of impotence are resolved by these simple changes.

Impotence is often the side effect of a prescription drug. According to the UCLA <u>Health Insights</u>, sixteen of the top 200 prescription drugs can cause impotence as a side effect. Many drugs prescribed for high blood pressure, like diuretics (nicknamed water pills), and Tagamet®, an anti-ulcer drug, can cause impotence. Any man who suddenly develops impotence while on a prescription medication should contact his physician immediately. Having your doctor change your drugs may eliminate the problem.

Any prolonged physical disease can cause impotence in a man, especially kidney disease or a disease that affects male hormone secretion.

Abuse of alcohol or drugs can cause impotence.

Impotence can be caused by psychological reasons: stress, fear of not being able to perform sexually, fear of causing unwanted pregnancy, worries about the relationship between the sex partners, problems with the man's feelings about sexuality, and being afraid of sex after surgery, fear of having a heart attack or other major health problems. The best ways to treat the psychological disorders is with professional counseling and learning how to properly deal with stress.

A mild stimulant, like caffeine in coffee, sometimes will help reduce impotence.

Indigestion
Indigestion or heartburn during the night can be caused by eating too close to the time you lie down to sleep. Doctors recommend that people should not eat for two to three hours before bedtime. While you're sleeping, all of your body functions slow down. The stomach does not digest food as quickly as usual, and too much stomach acid is produced. Because you are lying down while sleeping, some of the excess acid can "back up" and cause irritation in the stomach and esophagus. If you are regularly bothered by indigestion in the night, try raising the head of your bed by six inches. This

should create enough difference in the level of your head and your stomach so that the acid cannot flow up out of the stomach.

During the day, do not lie down if you are bothered by indigestion. Lying down just makes the problem worse. Sitting up or standing helps the stomach acids remain in the stomach. Also, avoid bending over. This puts more pressure on your abdomen, which can aggravate the indigestion.

Chocolate, peppermint, tobacco of any kind, aspirin, coffee, tea, fried foods, tomato products, onion, garlic, citrus fruits and juices, spicy or fatty foods can all cause indigestion and should be avoided if possible.

Develop good eating habits. Eat slowly by putting your knife and fork down between bites. This will slow down your eating and reduce the amount of air you swallow with each bite. It will allow your brain to notice how much food you are eating, and you will tend to eat less. Since much indigestion is caused by overeating, eating smaller meals will help reduce the problem.

Losing weight, especially around your waist, may be helpful in reducing the amount of indigestion you experience. Do not wear tight clothes, girdles or belts. Excess weight or tight clothing around the stomach puts extra pressure on it and can cause indigestion. Many women experience indigestion problems during pregnancy because of the extra pressure on their stomachs.

Folk medicine remedies include eating alfalfa sprouts or slices of raw potato or turnip to relieve indigestion. Drink lots of water. Avoid carbonated drinks, since they usually contain acid. Use caution in taking chewable or liquid antacids, since their frequent use can cause the stomach to actually produce more acid.

Some prescription and over-the-counter drugs, including aspirin and ibuprofen, can cause indigestion. If you are taking any medicine, discuss your indigestion problem with your doctor, and try to reduce or eliminate taking any drugs that might be causing the trouble.

Infertility

The inability to have children is a condition that more and more couples are facing. A woman is generally most fertile during the first half of her child-bearing years. Since more women are postponing having children until after the age of 30, the likelihood increases of their having problems getting pregnant. A serious, usually untreatable condition called endometriosis is often found in women over 30 who have never had children. This ailment causes infertility, because the normal functioning and placement of the tissue which lines the inner part of the uterus (the endometrium) is altered; the tissue actually grows out of the inner womb, often into the Fallopian tubes and even onto the ovaries.

There are several other causes of infertility, which are products of the Sexual Freedom Revolution. With the growing acceptance of sex-on-demand, venereal disease has increased dramatically. One of the consequences of VD in women is scar tissue on the reproductive organs. Such scarring can reduce or eliminate chances of conception or child-bearing. Further, widespread use of "artificial" contraceptives over the past 20 years has resulted in unexpected infertility problems. Oral contraceptives ("the pill") interfere with the normal hormone levels in a woman. Long-term use of the pill has left many women either temporarily or permanently infertile. Also, several kinds of intrauterine devices (IUD's), which are placed inside the womb to prevent the fertilized egg from implanting, have caused permanent damage to thousands of women.

A third result of the sex-without-responsibility era has been the fertility problems experienced by women who have had abortions — particularly those who've had more than one abortion. During an abortion procedure, the delicately thin wall of the uterus can easily, accidentally be punctured. This can result in severe scarring or even provoke endometriosis. Furthermore, if all the fetal tissue (that is, fingers, toes, hands, etc. of the unborn child) is not completely removed in an abortion, uterine problems can arise. Many times, excessive bleeding following an abortion results in the total removal of the uterus.

It should be recognized, however, that the problem of infertility has plagued many "innocent" couples for thousands of years. Men, as well as women, can have fertility difficulties. The same medical technology that has inadvertently caused some new types of infertility problems in this generation has also made great advances in treating infertility. There are numerous tests available to detect the cause(s) of infertility. New drugs and delicate surgical procedures have enabled many couples to become parents.

Couples trying to have children, who do not suspect any medical reasons for infertility, should first try the "Basal Body Temperature" method to determine when, and if, the woman is ovulating. Once ovulation is confirmed, the temperature system is a good way to try to time the fertilization of the egg (through natural intercourse) at the time of ovulation, the most likely time for conception.

Usually, a woman's temperature will remain fairly constant for the first two weeks of the cycle, then go up for the last two weeks. Ovulation is determined when a temperature change of .4 to .6°F occurs within a 24-hour time period, somewhere toward the end of the first 2-week period. There will usually be a slight decrease in temperature the day before ovulation and an increase the day after. Charting the body temperature and using it for family planning is known as the "Basal Body Temperature" method.

To determine ovulation, a woman should chart her daily temperature every morning before getting out of bed, drinking, eating, smoking or other physical activity. Using a "basal" thermometer with a widely spaced Fahrenheit scale, she should take her temperature for five minutes each morning. The daily temperatures should be recorded on a chart, which also notes the days of intercourse, days of menstruation, days of illness like cold or flu, any medication taken, or any other unusual situation. By keeping temperature charts for several months, and determining the normal ovulation cycle, intercourse just before the time ovulation is expected to occur should be most productive.

Recently, a study at the University of Texas, published in the Journal of the American Medical Association (JAMA 249: 2747) indicated that vitamin C may increase fertility in males by preventing the clumping of sperm, leaving more sperm available for fertilization. In a case of vitamin C deficiency, the sperm are clumped together and are unable to separate to swim towards the ovum and fertilize the egg. Men, especially smokers, who are prone to have a vitamin C deficiency, are recommended to take 500 milligrams of vitamin C for at least two weeks.

Extra vitamin C also may be needed by women who have taken oral contraceptives and are now trying to have children.

Vitamin B12 is important in maintaining fertility. Adult males and females need 3.0 micrograms of vitamin B12 daily.

Low rates of fertility, miscarriages and birth defects have been linked to deficiency of the mineral manganese. Adult men and women need 15 milligrams of manganese daily, according to the U.S. RDA (Recommended Daily Dietary Allowance). Manganese generally is deficient in the American diet.

Choline, a vitamin found in lecithin, soybeans, eggs, liver, wheat germ, fish, green vegetables, peanuts, brewer's yeast, and sunflower seeds, may also play a role in fertility. A study shows that choline supplements in food can increase the sizes of litters in some farm animals.

Zinc supplements and vitamin E supplements have been reported to reduce infertility. Adult men and women need 15 mg. of zinc daily, according to the U.S. RDA. The RDA for vitamin E is: adult males 12-15 I.U.; adult females 12 I.U.; pregnant women 15 I.U.; nursing mothers 16 I.U.

Insect Bites and Stings

If the bitten or stung person knows or suspects an allergy to insect bites or stings, get professional medical help immediately. Swelling, hives, rapid heartbeat, difficult breathing, feelings of faintness or shock are symptoms that medical treatment may be necessary.

Apply a paste of baking soda and vinegar or baking soda and witch hazel directly to the insect bite. It will help relieve itching and help the bite heal. Calamine lotion, products containing alcohol or benzocaine or antihistamine drugs will also help reduce the itching.

Pediatrics (68:744) journal recommends ice compresses and meat tenderizer to relieve the pain of bee stings. Applying ice while the person is lying down will reduce the swelling and lessen the pain. Lying down will help slow the circulation and reduce spreading of the toxic venom. The meat tenderizer seems to work because it contains the enzyme papain. Papain tenderizes meat by breaking down the tough meat fibers, and it breaks down the bee venom the same way, the journal says. Meat tenderizers are also recommended to relieve jellyfish stings and common insect bites.

Tea, coffee or caffeinated soft drinks may help to counteract the effects of insect stings. Alcohol dilates or enlarges blood vessels and may intensify the effects of insect stings by speeding up the circulation of venom.

Antiperspirants can be used to stop the itching of insect bites. Dermatology professor Dr. R. B. Rees, Jr. from the University of California at San Francisco explains that the skin is dried by the aluminum in antiperspirants. Drying the skin helps reduce the itching and inflammation caused by the insect bite.

Pastes of salt, baking soda, aspirin, or tobacco applied directly to skin around the bee sting should draw the venom of the sting out within five minutes, according to the University of Georgia College of Agriculture. The wet paste should be left on the bee sting for at least 30 minutes to be most effective. Many people, including columnist Ann Landers, have found that placing a raw onion on a bee sting or insect sting will help draw out the venom. Although there isn't any scientific proof for this theory, onions were used on bee stings and wasp stings by the Dakota and Winnebago Indians. However, if you have sensitive skin, the onion treatment may be too harsh for you.

Some people believe certain herbal scents, including garlic, citronella, vitamin B1 (thiamine), mint, orange or oil of pennyroyal will repel insects.

Dress appropriately when you are going to be outside. Always wear shoes and socks. Expose as little skin as possible by wearing long-sleeve shirts, full-length pants and a hat. Wear drab colored or white clothing. Avoid bright colors and floral prints, because insects are attracted to clothes that imitate flowers.

Don't stir up stinging insects by swatting at them. Remain calm and slowly walk away.

When walking outside, try to avoid flowers, flower beds, flowering trees, shrubs, fruit-bearing trees and other plants that attract bees and insects. Be particularly careful after a rain, or on bright, warm days wnen bees are more likely to sting. Avoid water spots, birdbaths or areas of standing water.

Before eating outdoors, thoroughly spray the picnic area with insect repellent. Keep all food well covered, and stay away from the trash cans.

Don't wear perfume, cologne, scented powder, deodorants or suntan lotions when outdoors. Be careful when exercising outside, because the odor of perspiration can attract insects.

Use air-conditioning whenever possible in your car or home, so that you can keep the windows closed and the insects out. Inspect the windows, screens and seals around your house, and repair any small holes or gaps where unwanted insects could enter.

Insomnia
Insomnia or loss of sleep is often caused by

drinking beverages or taking drugs containing caffeine. If you suffer from insomnia, try to avoid coffee, cola or pepper drinks, tea, chocolate and other beverages containing caffeine or at least drink them only in the morning. Modern Medicine (52: 145) reports that over 100 commonly used over-the-counter drugs and 65 prescription drugs contain caffeine. If you suffer from insomnia, you should check with your pharmacist or doctor about the prescription and over-the-counter drugs you are taking. Alternatives without caffeine can probably be found for you.

Quit smoking! Studies have shown that smokers have a more difficult time getting to sleep than non-smokers.

Magnesium chloride supplements may be an answer to beat insomnia, based on a study at the University of Pretoria in South Africa. Two hundred insomnia patients were able to fall asleep easily after taking magnesium supplements. By taking magnesium supplements all day, even patients who had relied on sleeping pills were able to fall asleep. They were more alert the next day, and they could be awakened during the night, if needed, and still fall back asleep. One of the bad effects of sleeping pills or other such medication is that the sleep that is induced is often so deep that people who take them can't be awakened in an emergency.

Making a concentrated effort to relax before

going to bed may help your sleeping habits. Reading a boring or calming book or magazine, watching pleasant programs on TV, taking a warm bath, or listening to gentle music may help to put you in the proper frame of mind for sleeping.

Try to go to bed at the same time each night. A regular sleep time will help to improve the quality of your sleep.

Lose weight. Interruptions in your breathing while asleep can wake you up. These sleep apneas may be eliminated or reduced by weight loss.

Practice relaxation methods once you are in bed trying to sleep. Everyone has heard about "counting sheep", or similar visualization of something repetitive, and it works, because it relaxes your mind, while avoiding distracting or disturbing thoughts. Don't think of work, the things you dind't get done that day, or all the things you have to do tomorrow. Think of peaceful things so you can help yourself relax. Try concentrating on consciously slowing down your breathing. Try relaxing parts of your body, starting with your toes and working your way up to your neck muscles and your head as you count backwards from 100.

The Contemplative Brothers produce a prayerful, nondenominational, Christian relaxation tape, "Insomnia", which works wonders to help people get to sleep. To order, send $10.00 to Contemplative Tapes, Box 8065, Columbus, Georgia 31908.

Many people wake up early in the night and can't get back to sleep. Most things that help induce sleep don't seem to work for these insomniacs. But doctors at Sleep Disorder Centers across the United States are now recommending therapy called sleep restriction. Therapy starts by first allowing only a little sleep, let's say 3 hours per night. Then, by adding 15 minutes more sleep each night, you can gradually reach your optimal amount of nightly sleep. Keep a journal of how much and how long you sleep. Use an alarm clock to make sure you increase the amount of sleep by only 15 minutes nightly. Once you reach your optimal level, sleeping through the night should be routine.

Dealing with a child who has problems sleeping requires special attention from the parents. Children should be taught good sleep habits early in life. If your children are having problems sleeping, you can help by establishing a regular bedtime and bedtime routine. This should be a quiet time that includes reading and prayers. Like adults, children shouldn't participate in any physical activity within an hour of bedtime, and they shouldn't watch any TV shows or movies that would cause them to become excited. Use a soft night-light or quiet radio music to help set the scene for peaceful sleep.

Don't make the bedroom a place of punishment by sending children to their rooms. If they associate their bedrooms with punishment, they will consider sleeping to be a form of punishment. If the child complains about being afraid, don't say there is nothing to be afraid of, but comfort the child and help the child to deal with that fear, acknowledging that it is a real fear that could cause many hours of lost sleep.

Kidney Disease

Studies of mice at Massachusetts General Hospital and the National Institutes of Health show that a diet high in omega-3 fatty acids (fish oils) may help prevent kidney disease. However, this is a very small study, and since it wasn't a study on human beings, do not rush out and take fish oil supplements based on this test. Nutritionists, however, are recommending incorporating more fish into our regular diet, by eating fish at least twice a week. Salmon, mackerel, tuna, sardines, crab, shrimp, lobster and other shellfish are all high in the beneficial omega-3 fatty acids.

Leg Cramps

Cramps in the calf muscles of the legs can be extremely painful, especially at night.

If leg cramps occur, stretching the legs may provide quick relief. While in bed, grab the toes and the ball of the foot and pull them forward until the cramps stop. Massaging the legs, wrapping the legs in warm towels, or putting the feet into cold water may help relieve the cramps.

Many people find relief from leg cramps by blowing into a paper bag — or even into CUPPED hands— then closing the mouth and letting the air come back into the nose for a count of 10 or more. Don't stretch your legs after the breathing procedure just described. This procedure takes just a couple of minutes for quick relief in most cases, even with repetitions.

Quinine sulfate can relieve the pain of night leg cramps and help relax the leg muscles. It is available over-the-counter in Quintrol®, Q-Vel®, Legatrin® and as generic quinine sulfate. Quinine should not be used by pregnant women. It can cause undesirable side effects like ringing in the ears, headaches or nausea.

Frequent exercising to stretch the calf muscles, by leaning forward and pressing up against a wall with your hands while keeping your heels on the floor, can help prevent leg cramps from occurring. Slowly stretch the calf muscles, at least three times each day, until the cramps stop occurring. Exercise these muscles often to help keep the cramps from starting again.

Leg cramps occur most often when the feet and toes are pointed. So, if you are bothered by leg cramps, try sleeping on your side or make a special effort not to point your toes while sleeping. If you sleep on your back, try propping up the covers with a board or a pillow, so the weight of the sheets is off your toes. Sleeping on your back with a small pillow under your knees or loosely wrapping your legs in towels each night may help prevent the cramps. Some doctors recommend elevating the foot of the bed about nine inches to prevent leg cramps (<u>Lancet</u> 1:203).

Memory Loss
Memory loss and mental confusion have been associated with a deficiency of thiamine (vitamin B1). Yeast, liver, whole-grain products, wheat, eggs, milk, nuts, potatoes, leafy green vegetables, kidney beans and seeds are natural sources of thiamine.

Choline is thought to improve memory in normal people. Although not proven, Alzheimer's disease, a disease affecting the memory in elderly people, may be slowed by supplementing the diet with lecithin. Choline and inositol are vitamin constituents of lecithin, which can be synthesized in the body. Therefore, supplementing choline and inositol or lecithin in the diet may also help improve the memory. Choline is naturally found in soybeans, eggs, fish, liver, wheat germ, green vegetables, peanuts, brewer's yeast and sunflower seeds. Inositol is naturally found in organ meats, yeast, beans, wholegrain products, peanuts and citrus fruits.

Doing crossword puzzles and word games can help older people retain their sense of reasoning, according to researchers at the University of Washington. They discovered that memory and reasoning often suffered when elderly minds were not actively used. Crossword puzzles and word games help to challenge the mind.

Also see: **Alzheimer's Disease.**

Menstrual Cramps

Many women experience varying degrees of cramps just before or at the beginning of their monthly menstruation. Simple home remedies can provide some relief: placing a hot water bottle or heating pad on the pelvic area, soaking in a hot bath, lying on your back with your knees bent, or lying on your side while curled up in the "fetal" position.

Some researchers believe that calcium and magnesium supplements, taken just prior to the monthly period, help to reduce cramps and premenstrual tension. Calcium levels are greatly affected by female hormone levels, which change radically during the menstrual cycle. Increasing the absorption of calcium just prior to menstruation should help.

In some cases, menstrual cramps are aggravated by a weak pelvic muscle, the pubococcygeus or PC muscle. This problem can be helped by simple exercises before monthly menstruation. Research has shown that by exercising the muscles for just 15 minutes each day, recurring menstrual cramps, urinary incontinence (a "leaky" bladder), and urinary tract infections can be reduced. As a pleasant side effect, PC exercises increase the likelihood of a woman experiencing orgasm during intercourse, and the same exercises increase sexual endurance for men by 50%, according to Dr. William E. Hartman and Marilyn Fithian at the Center for Marital and Sexual Studies in Long Beach, California.

For complete information on how to perform these simple exercises, please refer to: **PC EXERCISES** under **Urinary Incontinence.**

Menstrual Irregularities

Menstrual cycles may vary from 21 to 35 days. Twenty-eight (28) days is normal for about 50% of women. Variations from 28 days usually doesn't signal a problem if the cycle is regular. However, if several periods are skipped or if they are irregular in flow or length, a gynecologist should be consulted.

Absence of menstruation is called amenorrhea. Amenorrhea before the menopause can be caused by many factors: extreme weight gain or weight loss, improper nutrition, overexertion, hypothyroidism, stress, intensive athletic training, jet lag, prescription or over-the-counter drugs, serious illness or surgery, and hormone changes.

To resume the normal menstruation pattern, the cause of the problem must be discovered and treated. For example, if poor nutrition is suspected, the woman should begin a supervised nutrition plan.

Irregular menstruation may be caused by endometriosis, a condition where the tissue from the uterus starts to grow outside the inner lining of the womb. Endometriosis is a common problem for women who have postponed childbearing beyond the early and middle reproductive years.

Endometriosis can cause infertility and tumors. The risk of having endometriosis can be reduced by moderate exercise according to researchers at Harvard University. The study showed that women who began regular, moderate exercise programs, not Olympic-style or "marathon" training, had less risk of developing endometriosis. Training that is too strenuous can lead to total loss of menstruation.

Migraine Headaches: See **Headaches**

Morning Sickness

Morning sickness of pregnancy can sometimes be relieved or controlled with simple, natural methods. Eating soda crackers or dry popcorn may help relieve morning sickness. Don't eat or drink fast. Take small bites and sips slowly to avoid swallowing air. Some doctors recommend taking 50 mg. of vitamin B6 three or four times each day, but large doses of this vitamin may cause birth defects. Vitamin B6 was one of the two ingredients in the anti-morning sickness drug, Bendectin®, which was taken off the market because it might cause birth defects. Eating alfalfa sprouts, slices of raw potato or turnip to relieve nausea is an old folk remedy.

During the day, do not lie down if you are bothered by indigestion or nausea. Lying down often makes the problem worse. Sitting up or standing allows the stomach acids to remain in the stomach. Also, avoid bending over. This puts more pressure on your abdomen and can aggravate the nausea.

Chocolate, peppermint, tobacco of any kind, aspirin, coffee, tea, fried foods, tomato products, onion, garlic, rich foods, alcohol, strong odors, citrus fruits and juices, spicy or fatty foods can all aggravate indigestion. They should be avoided if possible.

If nausea and vomiting persist during pregnancy, see your doctor. Too much vomiting will rob your baby of the nutrition it needs to develop.

Motion Sickness

Motion sickness, including dizziness, nausea and vomiting, is caused when you are experiencing motion but your brain is not able to compensate for the motion. If you can see the motion you are experiencing, it will help you balance the sensations of movement received in your inner ears.

Some people are more sensitive to motion than others. If you know you are sensitive, you should plan your traveling carefully. Try to travel when you know you can stop and take a break from the constant movement. When traveling by car, either drive or ride in the front seat. If you are riding, look ahead, keep your eyes on the road and do not watch the scenery going past you on either side. If you are in a boat, stay on the deck and watch the land or the horizon. If you are flying, sitting over a wing may be best.

Before you travel, eat a light meal. If you don't eat at all, your blood sugar levels may fluctuate and increase your chances of motion sickness. Avoid smoking or tobacco smoke, strong odors, eating rich foods or drinking alcohol.

In a recent study, powdered ginger was highly effective in preventing motion sickness.

Osteoporosis

Osteoporosis is a serious loss and weakening of

the bone that affects women mostly after menopause, although men and younger women can also
suffer from it. Osteoporosis is often first noticed
because of a fracture of the hip, wrist or vertebrae
of the spine. Hip fractures are life-threatening in
the elderly. Within three months of a hip fracture,
15% of old people will die, often because of blood
clots that form in the legs during bed rest and then
break off and lodge in the lungs. Osteoporosis can
also cause loss of height, a humped back (often
called Dowager's hump) and extreme pain. Early
osteoporosis is difficult to diagnose, because you
cannot notice the gradual loss of bone as it happens.

Osteoporosis is usually noticed only after a great
amount of bone mass is lost, and fractures or perio-
dontal disease (gum disease) as a result of the deterioration of jaw bone start occurring. Therefore, it
is important to know who is at greatest risk, what
steps to take to prevent its development and what to
do if it occurs.

People at the greatest risk of losing their bone
mass and developing osteoporosis, are:

- women
- Caucasians
- people with translucent or very fair skin
- cigarette smokers
- people who suffer from anorexia nervosa, a
  drastic loss of appetite

- people with a slender build
- inactive people
- women who are past menopause
- people who consume large amounts of caffeine
- people with a family history of osteoporosis or hip fractures
- people who have taken long-term treatment with steroid drugs for arthritis, asthma or other diseases
- people who drink lots of soft drinks
- people who eat high protein diets
- people who consume large amounts of alcohol

Damage from osteoporosis usually is permanent. The only treatment is heat, drugs for the pain, a back brace and rest. Rest, combined with moderate exercise like walking, helps keep the muscles in shape to support the weak bone structure.

Since damage from osteoporosis cannot be cured, prevention should be a life-long goal. Women who have any of the risk factors listed above, any of them, should work actively to protect themselves against osteoporosis. It is often difficult to convince a woman in her prime that her lifestyle will affect the strength of her bones and the quality of her health after menopause — but it is essential. Some of the risk factors, like family history or individual bone structure, are things we cannot change, but some things can be changed. The first step in prevention is to eliminate the unnecessary risks: quit smoking and reduce the intake of caffeine, soft drinks, meat, high protein foods and alcohol.

Consuming adequate, but not excessive, calcium and vitamin D is important in prevention. Dr. Morris Notelovitz, M.D., Ph.D., author of Stand Tall the definitive book on osteoporosis, recommends 800 - 1,000 milligrams of calcium daily (for women prior to menopause) and 1,200 to 1,400 milligrams (for women after menopause). The best way to get daily calcium is from foods like milk, cheese, nuts, tofu and leafy, green vegetables. Three eight-ounce glasses of milk a day should supply your needs. If you don't like milk or need to supplement your diet, calcium carbonate is usually recommended. However, calcium carbonate may cause gas problems in some people, so calcium citrate, lactate or gluconate can be used. It doesn't matter if the source is oyster shells, "all-natural", or in a fancy bottle, as long as it is calcium. The important thing to watch is how much "elemental calcium" is available. The least expensive generic brand of calcium is fine and will be the most cost effective. Antacids like Tums®, which have only calcium carbonate as an active ingredient, are often cheaper than other calcium supplements. If you use calcium supplements, take them throughout the day, rather than all at once, so the calcium will be best absorbed by the body. Bonemeal is NOT recommended as a good source of calcium, because its high lead content can cause liver or kidney damage.

Anyone with kidney stones or kidney problems should NOT take calcium or increase their intake of calcium rich foods unless their physician agrees.

Substances found in food, including oxalic acid (found in rhubarb and spinach), phosphorus (found in soft drinks and in many other foods), phytic acid (found in whole-grain products), corticosteroid drugs (such as cortisone and prednisone), dilantin, anticonvulsant drugs, tobacco, alcohol, caffeine or an excessive amount of protein in the diet can interfere with calcium absorption or cause the body to need more calcium.

Researchers at the University of Chicago Medical Center have discovered that glucose polymer, a type of sugar made from cornstarch, may help people absorb and retain more calcium. Although glucose polymer is now available in syrup or dried forms, more research is needed to discover its role in the prevention of osteoporosis.

Exercise helps prevent osteoporosis. Studies have shown that weight-bearing exercise helps the bones to grow stronger and more dense, so there is less chance of developing osteoporosis later on. Weight-bearing exercise is an activity like aerobics, dancing, walking, jogging, rowing, hiking, ope jumping, tennis or bicycling, where the bones have to support body weight. Swimming is not a "weight-bearing" exercise, since the water supports the body while swimming. It is good for an aerobic work-out and developing muscle strength, but not for developing bone strength.

Excessive exercise actually can cause osteoporosis. Women who have a very rigorous training schedule sometimes stop menstruating. This is a severe risk for osteoporosis, since the hormone levels in the body are altered. Training should be balanced so the menstrual cycle and hormonal balance are maintained.

"Estrogen replacement is the single most effective means of preventing osteoporosis," writes Vivian Lewis, M.D. of the University of Illinois College of Medicine. Other studies, including one by Linda S. Richelson, M.P.H. in the New England Journal of Medicine (311: 1273-5), have also explained that the loss of estrogen after menopause or removal of the ovaries, rather than the aging process, is responsible for most of the bone loss leading to osteoporosis in women. The FDA and the National Institutes of Health (NIH) advisory panel say that estrogen helps the absorption and retention of calcium by the bones. Minimal doses of estrogen and progestin seem to have the best results with the fewest side effects. Estrogen replacement therapy should start immediately following menopause, either natural menopause or when the ovaries are surgically removed. When estrogen replacement therapy is started right after women stop menstruating, hip and wrist fractures can be reduced as much as 60%, according to the NIH.

Estrogen replacement therapy is only available by prescription and while under a physician's supervision. Estrogen should not be used, or used cautiously, by women with heart disease, high blood pressure, endometriosis, asthma, epilepsy, diabetes, severe migraine headaches, gallstones, breast or uterine cancer, family history of cancer or gallbladder problems.

Vitamin D is needed to help the body properly use and absorb calcium; thus, both are vital to bone health. However, according to Dr. Lewis, only the U.S. Recommended Daily Allowance (RDA) of 200-400 International Units (I.U.) is required. Many people get enough vitamin D in sunshine and their regular diet. Vitamin D is also naturally found in fish, liver, eggs and artificially in fortified milk. Do not take excessive supplements of vitamin D, because it is fat soluble, can stay in the body for a long time, and can cause side effects when taken in doses just larger than the RDA. However, the need for vitamin D increases as you grow older, because the body does not absorb it as readily.

Magnesium is an essential mineral that works with calcium and phosphorus to form bone. Whole-grain products, vegetables, seafood and peanuts are good sources of magnesium. The U.S. Recommended Daily Allowance (RDA) of magnesium for adult women is 300 mg.

Molybdenum is an often overlooked trace mineral which can help prevent osteoporosis. Unfortunately, it is often deficient in the American diet. Supplements containing 30 to 100 <u>microg</u>rams can supply enough for strong bones.

Fluoride may help increase bone density. Studies are now underway at the Mayo Clinic in Rochester, Minnesota and other institutions to see what level of fluoride is the best for prevention of osteoporosis and how fluoride treatment may help the absorption of calcium and other necessary minerals. (<u>Annals</u> <u>of</u> <u>Internal</u> <u>Medicine</u> 98:1013). However, fluoride may cause dangerous side effects, and supplementation should only be done under a doctor's supervision.

Being safety conscious may help prevent undue stress and strain on the joints, especially for women past menopause with any of the risk factors for osteoporosis. Wearing low-heeled shoes, avoiding hazardous weather conditions and simply being careful may help prevent the fractures of osteoporosis from occurring.

Pain
The higher your blood sugar is, the less able you

are to tolerate pain, according to research at the University of Minnesota College of Medicine, published in The American Journal of Medicine (77: 79). Since diabetics must be vigilant to keep their blood-sugar levels low, this is an especially important discovery for them. Generally, diabetics were found to have a lower tolerance for pain than non-diabetics. Other studies have shown that high blood-sugar levels reduce the effect of narcotic drugs prescribed for pain. Keeping blood sugar counts at low, acceptable levels will help diabetics to tolerate pain better.

Individuals feel pain differently, according to Dr. Arthur Barsky, an assistant psychiatry professor at Harvard Medical School. Dr. Barsky says that circumstances, attention and mood affect how many people feel pain. For example, soldiers wounded during World War II felt less pain from their injuries than people in the United States who had received the same wounds. Because the soldiers felt they had received the wounds while defending their country, their pain didn't seem as great. Although we can't usually affect the circumstances that cause pain, Dr. Barsky points out that we can alter our approach to pain. Pain does not seem as severe if we remain calm and avoid becoming anxious or depressed. Many techniques taught at childbirth classes are based on this approach of facing pain with calmness.

Dr. Arnold Fox of the University of California at Irvine claims that an amino acid can reduce pain in about 80 percent of the general population. The amino acid is DLPA, short for d,l,phenylalanine. It is available in many health food stores and some drugstores. Dr. Fox recommends taking 375 to 400 milligrams of DLPA with each meal to reduce the pain of arthritis, migraine headaches, back problems, and depression. DLPA has few known side effects and seems to work by stimulating the brain's neurohormones to block pain signals, according to the doctor.

Poison Ivy And Poison Oak

The best way to deal with the pain and itching of poison ivy or poison oak is to cleanse the area with plain soap and water or rubbing alcohol immediately after you have come in contact with either of the plants. Repeat the cleaning process three times to be sure that all of the plant's oil is removed from the skin. If you have touched the plants with your hands or suspect that they have been contaminated by touching your clothes, scrub your hands and clean thoroughly under your fingernails.

If you are very sensitive to the poison ivy or poison oak plants, you can become infected just by contacting clothing, material (like tent fabric), tools or equipment that has been exposed to the plants. The allergic power of the plant can also be transmitted by an animal, like a family dog, that has contacted the plant. Contaminated pets, tools and materials should be thoroughly cleaned to remove possible contamination. Never burn the plants — but consider having a non-sensitive person remove any poison oak or poison ivy from your property. Smoke from burning poison oak or poison ivy can cause a severe allergic reaction, particularly in the eyes.

If the itching and inflammation of poison ivy or poison oak appear, try bathing in a hot tub of water with one cup of oatmeal or an oatmeal product called Aveeno®. Use moderately HOT water for all baths or showers, because moderately hot water releases the histamine in the skin's cells. Histamine causes the intense itching. Even though the hot water will cause itching while bathing, you will have hours of relief after the bath. Avoid using calamine lotion in the early stages of eruptions, since the calamine lotion can actually spread the oil from poison ivy or poison oak. Do not scratch the sores, because scratching can spread the infection to other parts of the body.

Premenstrual Syndrome (PMS)

Premenstrual syndrome involves a variety of problems that women may experience immediately before monthly menstruation. For years, the symptoms of water retention, depression, weight gain, anxiety, irritability, headaches, dizziness, tender breasts and tiredness were not acknowledged by male physicians as a "real" problem. Only recently has the medical community started accepting the fact that PMS can be a mild aggravation for some women, yet be a serious and threatening experience for others.

Premenstrual fluid retention, weight gain, arthritis associated with female hormone deficiency, and symptoms of depression may be helped by taking vitamin B6 (pyridoxine) daily during premenstrual problems.

Anxiety, irritability, headaches, dizziness, cravings for sweets or chocolate, tender breasts, confusion and tiredness may be helped by supplements of vitamin E, B1, C, d,l,phenylalanine, magnesium, chromium, and zinc.

Current research indicates that 375 - 400 mg. supplements of d,l,phenylalanine provide amazing relief to chronic PMS sufferers. This amino acid has been found to be a substance in chocolate that causes many people to crave it. For maximum effectiveness, the supplements must be taken daily at mealtimes, for several weeks.

Some researchers believe that calcium and magnesium supplements taken just before the monthly period help to reduce cramps and premenstrual tension. Calcium levels are greatly affected by hormone levels, which change radically during the menstrual cycle. Increasing the absorption of calcium just before menstruation should help alleviate the irregularities.

Regulating the body's blood sugar level may help reduce PMS. Eating several small meals each day, including fresh fruits and vegetables, will help regulate the blood sugar better than eating only three meals a day.

To prevent excess fluid retention which may add to PMS problems, try the following: exercise regularly; lose weight; AVOID all salt; rest your legs and feet at least twice a day by lying with your feet higher than your heart; wear support panty-hose when possible. Avoid eating black licorice or products containing licorice extracts, because they may contribute to salt and fluid retention.

Psoriasis: See **Skin Problems**

Senility: See **Alzheimer's Disease** and **Memory Loss**

Skin Problems
If you suffer from dry skin or eczema, dress

lightly to avoid sweating. Perspiring increases dry skin problems. Do not wear clothes made from wool or silk, because these materials can aggravate dry skin. Whatever you do, DO NOT SCRATCH! Scratching will only irritate the skin and make the condition worse.

Wash only with cool or lukewarm water; hot water dries out the skin. Use a non-irritating soap that contains a moisturizer rather than a "pure" soap. Avoid using any gel or lotion that contains alcohol, because it will dry out the skin. Do not use bubble bath. According to the U.S. Food and Drug Administration, "Excessive use (of bubble bath) or prolonged exposure may cause irritation to skin and urinary tract. Discontinue use if rash, redness or itching occurs."

The U.S. Pharmacist (13-12:24) suggests soaking in warm water for about ten minutes when bathing. This will allow the water to penetrate deeply into the skin. After drying thoroughly, apply cream or ointment, which will act as a barrier to keep in the moisture that has just been absorbed by the skin. The skin should be gently, but thoroughly, dried by patting with a towel, not rubbing. If the skin is still wet on its surface, the lotion will not be able to provide complete protection. Moisturize your feet, toes and toe cuticles to help keep your feet from cracking and drying.

To prevent overdrying the skin in winter, try to

take fewer baths and more showers. If possible, take your bath or shower just before bed rather than in the morning. An evening bath will give your body the whole night to naturally replace the body's own oils and moisturizers.

Dry skin is extremely noticeable in the winter months when the air within the home is usually very dry. Adding a cool-air humidifier to your home will help. Also, growing plants that require a lot of water, like ferns or large-leaved plants like begonias and bamboo, will help because they give off moisture! Try placing some of these plants in your bedroom and around the house to add extra moisture to the air.

The best way to protect your skin from disease and signs of aging is to avoid excessive exposure to the sun. Skin cancer and little brown splotches known as aging spots are directly related to the ultraviolet rays of the sun. Sunbathers or people who spend a lot of time outdoors, or those who use sun lamps, are at the highest risk for these skin problems. You can lower your risk by ALWAYS using a sun screen, preferably with a SPF (sun protection factor) of 15, wearing protective sun glasses, hats, or visors while in the sun, avoiding direct sunlight between 10 am and 2 pm each day, and by wearing long-sleeves if you are driving for long distances in the summer with a car window down. Sitting under an umbrella at the beach may protect you from direct sunlight, but the dangerous rays bounce off the sand and back under the umbrella. Even under an umbrella, you should still protect your skin.

Psoriasis, a chronic skin disease that causes scaly red patches of skin on the arms, elbows, scalp, knees, legs, and other parts of the body, may be reduced by cutting arachidonic acid (AA) out of the diet. Arachidonic acid (AA) is found in meat, eggs, poultry and dairy products and has been found to cause the patches of psoriasis to turn red and swell according to the journal CUTIS (34:497). It is recommended that people suffering from psoriasis try a diet of fruit, vegetables, bread and other cereal products, and fish, to lessen the occurrences of psoriasis. Fish oil capsules are also reported to help neutralize the AA found in our diets.

Many people with skin problems, like eczema, wear rubber gloves when doing dishes and other chores to "protect" their hands. However, the chemicals in rubber gloves often bother people with sensitive skin, according to the journal Contact Dermatitis (14:20). Plastic gloves are a better choice. If possible, buy plastic gloves that are extra large, and wear a pair of cotton gloves underneath. The cotton gloves will help absorb sweat and protect your skin.

Women with skin that is easily irritated should be sure to keep their make-up applicators, including sponges, eye wands and puffs, very clean. Keeping these applicators extremely clean, or trying new ways to apply make-up, may help to relieve or control unnecessary skin irritation.

The Food and Drug Administration (FDA)'s Division of Cosmetic Technology says that moisturizers with exotic names like placental extracts, collagen or elastin are no more effective than grape seed oil, squalene (shark liver oil) or geranium oil. There is NOT ONE PRODUCT that can prevent or reverse the effects of aging, according to the FDA. Rather than expensive creams and store-made moisturizers, many models will use nothing but food shortening to keep their skin soft and smooth.

Shaving irritates skin. Never shave dry, according to experts at Schick interviewed in Family Circle. Lubricate the skin first, with shaving cream, warm water, soapy water, baby oil or olive oil. Moisturize your skin immediately after shaving with an alcohol-free moisturizer. Shaving can actually help keep your skin smooth by removing the dead layers of skin, but you must moisturize the shaved area and replace any lost moisture.

Puffy eyes and bags under the eyes can be relieved by placing slices of cold cucumbers or potatoes on the closed eyes. However, it seems that any kind of cold compress will work just as well. Some models place used tea bags on their eyes, because tea contains tannin that causes the skin to tighten up, but just temporarily. Tannin is thought to be a cancer-causing agent and can also stain the skin, so we cannot recommend tea bags. Sometimes puffy eyes in the morning can be caused by detergent in your bed sheets that is irritating your eyes. Try rinsing your sheets and pillow cases at least two extra times or switch to a mild soap instead of a detergent.

Chapped and dry lips are often relieved by a product like Chapstick® or Vaseline Petroleum Jelly®. However, be sure to only coat the red part of your lips with the balm. Petroleum based products clog the pores on your skin, and if you smear the balm on your skin, you may develop severe blackheads, pimples and skin problems in the area right around your lips. (<u>CUTIS</u> 37: 6,459).

Some people suffer from allergies to metals that cause their skin to become red, swollen and itchy. Allergies to nickel may occur with use of an ear-piercing instrument containing nickel. Be sure to have ear-piercing done with a sterilized and nickel-free stainless steel instrument. For some people, coating nickel-plated items with clear nail polish helps reduce irritation, but nickel should be avoided completely, if possible. If you suspect you have a nickel allergy, avoid any jewelry containing nickel, and any nickel-plated paper clips, car keys, or eye-lash curlers.

Seborrheic keratoses are often called "the barnacles of aging" and are the most common noncancerous skin tumors that affect older white Americans. Seborrheic keratoses are brown or yellow raised spots with a greasy, scaly crust that most often appear on the shoulders, back and upper chest. They can be scraped off by a doctor.

To prevent wrinkles, we should watch the way we speak and the way we sleep, says Samuel Stegman, a dermatologist from San Francisco. When talking, we often frown, tighten our lips and make other faces that help create wrinkles, Stegman says. He suggests placing a mirror by your telephone to see how you move your face, so you can develop better facial control. Pushing your head against your pillow when you sleep can cause wrinkles, too. Some wrinkles and skin creases are directly related to how people sleep, according to Stegman. To help prevent wrinkles, try to avoid pushing your head down into your pillow or mattresses.

Freckles, including "age spots", can be reduced or removed by a solution of lemon juice or buttermilk and oatmeal. Keep the solution on the skin for at least 10 minutes, and repeat this procedure each day until the freckles fade.

Sleep Problems: See Insomnia

Smoking — How To Quit

"Cigarette smoking is the single largest preventable cause of disease and death in the United States," according to the American College of Obstetricians and Gynecologists. Over 41,000 Americans die every year as a result of cigarette smoking. Smoking increases chances of getting emphysema, bronchitis, heart attacks, strokes, or cancer of the lungs, mouth, bladder, pancreas, larynx or esophagus. Women who smoke are more likely to develop osteoporosis, give birth to a dead baby, have a miscarriage or deliver a low-birth-weight baby, when pregnant.

As well as reducing your risks of long-term health problems, there are immediate benefits to quitting smoking. You will be able to breathe more easily, and you'll find you have greater endurance when participating in sports activities. Your senses of taste and smell improve. The stains on your hands and your teeth disappear, and your breath gets sweeter. After you quit, you will have fewer colds, and within two weeks you should notice an improvement in your "smoker's hack" or cough.

The first step to quitting is discovering why you smoke. Do you feel that smoking relaxes you and calms your nerves? Do you smoke just to "fit in" the crowd? Do you think of smoking as a pleasure that you give yourself? Whatever the reason, you must convince yourself that you can achieve it without smoking. Deciding to quit and taking the responsibility for your smoking are very important. Only you can make this life-changing decision.

You will need the support of your friends and loved ones when you decide to quit. This time will be difficult, and you will need their patience and help. There is a definite physical addiction to the nicotine found in cigarettes, and breaking that addiction is often the most difficult part of quitting.

Withdrawal from nicotine can be eased by a prescription drug called Nicorette® which slowly releases a measured dose of nicotine into the system to reduce physical craving for tobacco products. Withdrawal from nicotine may also be eased by taking half a teaspoon of bicarbonate of soda in a glass of water two or three times a day. Apparently, the bicarbonate of soda helps hold nicotine in the system and reduce withdrawal symptoms by giving the body more time to adapt to withdrawal.

Once a smoker has successfully withdrawn from tobacco for two weeks, most withdrawal symptoms should pass.

Regular, aerobic exercise, such as running, walking, playing tennis, swimming, bike riding, hard physical labor, and association with non-smokers help in giving up smoking and resisting temptation to return to smoking.

Snoring

Snoring can be aggravating to a sleeping partner, as well as harmful to the sleeper. Since many people snore only when they lie flat on their backs and their jaws drop open, try this simple suggestion. In the top of the snorer's pajamas, sew in a large fishing sinker, golf ball, marble or other hard, round object, as suggested by an article in <u>Southern</u> <u>Medical</u> journal (79:1061). The object should be sewn in so that if the snorer rolls onto his back, the annoying object will press right on the spine below the neck. Then, the snorer will usually roll onto his side, without waking up!

Snoring is associated with a more dangerous sleep problem called sleep apnea — when someone stops breathing during sleep. Loud snoring or severe snoring episodes associated with gaps in breathing should be reported to your doctor.

Sores

Pressure sores or bed sores occur when a person must lie in bed for long periods of time, often during recuperation from a serious illness or accident. Stroke victims and people in comas frequently have sores develop in areas where the body has most pressure. In their initial stages, bed sores are just annoying, but left unnoticed or untreated, they can become serious problems that jeopardize the overall health of the patient.

Application of cod liver oil, castor oil, granulated sugar, ice packs, linseed oil, cornstarch, egg whites or honey have been recommended as home treatments for bed sores. Unfortunately, none of these methods has been proven to be effective. The most effective treatment for bed sores is to remove the pressure on the area and treat the sore with a local antibiotic.

Of course, it is best to <u>prevent</u> bed sores from occurring. A person who is forced to stay in bed for several days should be turned every two hours, when possible. Using a water mattress, air bed, lying on a sheep-skin pad or foam may help reduce pressure sores. Bed sheets should be kept loose, and the person should be kept dry. Excess sweating or incontinence increases the chances of pressure sores developing. Minimize raising the head of the bed, because more pressure is shifted to the lower part of the body where pressure sores often form.

Sore Throat: See **Throat Infections**

Stress

Stress can be very harmful to your health if you do not handle it properly. Stress can contribute to headaches, cramps, indigestion, nausea, allergies, tiredness, backaches, depression, stiff necks, ulcers, colitis and heart disease. Techniques for stress management should be appropriate for the kind of stress you are experiencing. Physical methods like deep breathing and exercise should be used to cope with physical reactions to stress, like body aches, hyperactivity and the jitters. Mental calming methods should be used for mental stress.

Be sure to take time for yourself. Relaxation away from the stresses and strains of demanding situations gives you time to unwind and rejuvenate your body and your emotional stability. Develop a hobby that you enjoy. If you are an avid art lover, take time for yourself and visit an art gallery. Having fun should be an integral part of your life.

Talk. Talk about your concerns, your fears, your dreams, your anxieties to your closest friend or spouse. Talking helps put the problems into correct perspective and helps the problem and the stress from becoming bottled up inside.

Don't be afraid to cry to release tension. Crying is one of our body's natural ways of dealing with stress. Dr. Louis M. Savary believes that groaning is another natural response to stress and pain. People who are hurt groan in an effort to deal with the pain and stress, says Dr. Savary. He believes that 10-20 minutes of groaning (preferably while lying on the floor in a dark room or while alone in the car) will help relieve stress.

Learn deep breathing techniques, read inspirational books or start an active prayer life. Take hot baths and massages.

Admit you are feeling stressed. Just as alcoholics must admit they have a problem before they can be treated, it is very important that stressed people admit they are suffering from stress before they can be helped.

Accept your own personal limitations. Accept the limitations of money. You will always want more than you have, and you may have to sacrifice some things to get what is important to you. Accept the limitations of your situation. If your plane is delayed or you are stuck in a traffic jam, worrying and getting angry will not make the situation disappear.

Some doctors, including Robert T. Johnson, M.D., author of <u>Stay Well</u>, recommend chamomile tea and the amino acid dietary supplement tryptophan as natural relaxants. .

Pleasant music, whatever kind of music you like, may be calming. Some people also believe that certain sounds are relaxing. You can buy tapes of "relaxing sounds" that include the sounds like gentle waves crashing on a shore. Experiment with the sounds that you find calming, both in music and in nature, and keep your environment conducive to relaxation. The Contemplative Brothers in Columbus, Georgia, sell relaxation tapes that have a prayerful, nondenominational Christian focus. For a price list write: Contemplative Tapes, Box 8065, Columbus, Georgia, 31908.

To ease mental stress, some doctors recommend visualization. The person visualizes the stressful situation and how to resolve the problem, therefore ending the tension. Visualizing a positive ending to the situation seems to help the person cope with the stress.

Dietary supplementation with vitamin C and iron, which is necessary for the formation of red blood cells which help carry oxygen to the body, may help fight stress. Stress may increase the need for niacin (Vitamin B3) and thiamine (Vitamin B1).

Chemists are now claiming that certain fragrances can help calm us in times of stress. Many cosmetics companies are marketing fragrance vials that contain "spiced apple" or other smells that are supposed to help us relax. In the South, pots of water containing special herbs and spices are kept on wood stoves, electric or gas ranges to create a special mood in the house. Research has proven that animals are greatly influenced by smells and aromas, but whether or not human beings can become relaxed just by breathing a certain scent is not known. However, if you have a certain aroma that you associate with peacefulness and calm, like the smell of hot apple pie baking in the oven, maybe fragrance therapy will help you relax.

The best way to prepare your body to cope with stress is to get plenty of rest (7 to 8 hours of sleep each night), exercise regularly, avoid eating foods high in fats or salt, and eat nutritious foods. Researchers in France, and Dr. Burton M. Altura of Brooklyn, New York, have discovered that low magnesium levels make it more difficult to deal with stress, so be sure to get between 300 and 400 milligrams of magnesium daily. Avoid cigarettes, alcohol, caffeine and any other substances that are harmful to the body. Plan to manage your stress as much as you can. Limit the number of life changes you make at one time; set realistic goals; take control over your environment by rearranging or redecorating your home or office; organize your workload; and discuss your problems with a friend or professional counselor.

When working with stress, try to remain open and flexible to new ideas. You will be better able to cope with the stress of the situation.

Stroke Prevention

A stroke occurs when a blood vessel in the brain ruptures or becomes blocked by a clot. Strokes are closely related to coronary heart disease and atherosclerosis, so things that help prevent them may also help prevent strokes.

Risk factors for stroke include smoking, being

overweight, having high blood pressure, hardening of the arteries, diabetes, meningitis, congenital heart disorders, sickle cell anemia, and taking oral contraceptives.

Therefore, to avoid a stroke: (1) maintain your ideal weight (2) do not smoke (3) keep blood pressure under control (4) lower blood cholesterol (5) practice stress reduction and learn how to cope with stress (6) exercise regularly.

If you are at high risk for a stroke, you may consider taking daily aspirin. Studies have shown that just a small amount of daily aspirin, as little as a baby aspirin or half a regular aspirin, may help to prevent strokes. DO NOT start this treatment without your doctor's consent, because it is NOT considered standard medical practice at this time. Don't take a lot of aspirin. Aspirin can cause bleeding, especially if taken in large doses.

Many people often suffer several small strokes without realizing that a stroke has occurred, according to Columbia University's Health and Nutrition newsletter. Without medical treatment, the strokes usually increase in severity, so it is important to recognize the early warning signs of stroke and get quick medical attention. Contact your doctor immediately if you notice: any paralysis on one side of your face or body, sudden loss of vision in just one eye, numbness or weakness on one side of your body or in one arm or leg, unusual and severe headaches, unusual dizziness or loss of ability to speak properly or to find the words you want to say.

Sunburn

The ultraviolet rays from the sun can be very dangerous and can cause skin cancer to appear later in life. It is very important that you try to protect yourself from sunburn, rather than trying to relieve sunburn once it has occurred.

Sunbathers and people who spend a lot of time outdoors, or those who use sun lamps need to be extremely careful. You can lower your risk of sunburn by wearing a sunscreen, long-sleeve tops and long pants, protective sun glasses, hats, or visors while in the sun. Sitting under an umbrella at the beach may protect you from direct sunlight, but the dangerous rays bounce off the sand and back under the umbrella. Even under an umbrella, you should still protect your eyes and wear a sunscreen to protect your skin.

If a minor sunburn does occur, here are some home remedies to help relieve the pain. Try gently rubbing the sunburn with cider vinegar. Soak your whole body in a bathtub of cool water which will help the skin release the heat. Apply a paste of baking soda and water (or baking soda and milk) directly to the affected area. Leave the paste on until the sunburn cools. Lotions or creams containing Benzocaine provide quick, effective relief.

Vitamin C is necessary for fast healing of sunburn. Taking extra vitamin C before or after receiving a sunburn is proven to help the healing process.

Tailbone Pain

Pain in the tailbone, medically called coccygodynia, can be disconcerting. Some people have a sharp pain, yet other people experience more of a constant dull pain.

The <u>Mayo</u> <u>Clinic</u> <u>Health</u> <u>Letter</u> points out that many teenagers suffer from this problem, because they wear tight, heavy jeans and sit on hard, uncomfortable school chairs for several hours each day. If you or someone you know has this problem, try wearing only loose-fitting, lightweight pants. Also, be sure to sit in comfortable, well-padded chairs as often as possible. Practice good posture when you are sitting or standing. This will often help relieve or eliminate tailbone pain.

Temporomandibular Joint (TMJ) Dysfunctions

Headaches, dental problems, ear aches, pain and numbness in the face, jaw, head, neck, upper arms, or spine can be caused by disorders of the temporomandibular (TMJ) joints. The temporomandibular joints are the jaw joints that you can feel near your ears as you open and close your mouth. The TMJ system also includes nearby teeth and many of the intricate muscles and ligaments that connect the joints.

Most TMJ problems cannot be cured, but they can be managed so they don't create so many long-reaching problems. Clenching or grinding your teeth can cause dislocation of the TM joints. Sometimes teeth clenching and grinding can be stopped by practicing relaxation techniques, but professional counseling may be necessary if the behavior is a result of deep tension or anxiety.

Many people suffering from TMJ dysfunctions have learned to relax their jaw joints by keeping their lips together but their teeth apart. This is the natural way for the jaw to rest, but many people try to force their teeth together, even when their lips are closed. Consciously relaxing the jaw joints may be all that is needed to stop the pain caused by the joint dysfunction.

If sharp facial or TMJ pain occurs, applying moist heat (like that from a hot water bottle) or ice may provide simple relief. Eat only soft foods so the jaw will not have to work very hard. Get as much sleep as possible. Rest will help the supporting muscles to relax and ease the strain on the jaw joints.

Throat Infections Or Soreness

Sore throats sometimes need to be treated with antibiotics, so check with your doctor before trying home treatment.

Keeping the throat moist is the best way to soothe the pain of a sore throat. Try drinking plenty of warm, sugar-free drinks or sucking on ice cubes made from sugar-free drinks.

Gargling with salt water (1/2 teaspoon of salt dissolved in 1/2 cup of warm water) will help to treat and soothe the throat infection. After the initial stinging from the gargling subsides, hot tea with honey is often recommended. Another suggestion is mixing 2 tablespoons of vinegar and 2 tablespoons of honey in one cup of lemon juice. Heat and drink the lemon, honey and vinegar combination. It relieves sore throats and helps clear up congestion for many people. Although this remedy is soothing, sugar in the honey may promote the growth of bacteria in the throat.

While fighting a sore throat, keep the air around you as moist as possible. Breathing moist air, like in a shower, steam from a kettle, a moist humidifier or vaporizer is an effective way to soothe sore throats. A humidifier in your bedroom may be the best way to fight recurring sore throats.

The American Academy of Otolaryngology —
Head and Neck Surgery reports that occasional sore
throats may be caused by regurgitating acids from
the stomach. When the stomach acid reaches the
back of the throat, it can be very irritating and
cause minor sore throat symptoms. To avoid this,
do not eat or drink within two hours before sleeping. The Academy also recommends tilting your
bed frame so the head of your bed is about six inches higher than the foot. Having your head higher
will make it difficult for the stomach acids to come
up and irritate the throat.

If you are trying to check a child for a sore throat,
try using a candy sucker instead of a tongue depres-
sor. It works wonders.

Disinfecting your toothbrush can kill the germs
that caused sore throats and can prevent you from
re-infecting yourself. Try disinfecting your toothbrush by soaking it in a dilute hydrogen peroxide
solution, then thoroughly rinsing the toothbrush
with water before using it.

Or, rather than trying to disinfect your toothbrush, some dentists recommend throwing it away
at the beginning signs of a cold or sore throat.
Then they advise disgarding that toothbrush as
soon as the throat infection is cleared up. Dr. Tom
Glass of the Oklahoma University School of Dentistry discovered that colds, sore throats, gum disease, mouth sores and some other infections keep

returning because the organisms are reproducing right on the toothbrush. During any infection in the mouth, Dr. Glass recommends using the same toothbrush for only one month. And remember, even when you are completely healthy, the American Dental Association recommends that you replace your toothbrush every three to four months.

To keep your neck warm while fighting off a sore throat, try tying a sock or scarf around your neck. It may look unusual, but as long as you're at home suffering with a cold, it shouldn't matter what you look like, as long as it works!

Ticks: Removing Woodticks and Other Ticks

If a woodtick is lodged in the skin of a person or animal, suffocate the tick by covering it with petroleum jelly, olive oil, mineral oil or nail polish. The tick will not be able to breathe and will remove its head from the body where it is lodged. Another trick that works is to touch the tick with a lighted cigarette or the hot head of a match that has just been blown out. Don't pull ticks off. When a tick is pulled off, the head of the tick often comes off and stays in the skin where it may cause infection.

Tinnitus: See Ear Noises

Tiredness: See Fatigue

Ulcers

Ulcers, which can be life threatening, should only be treated under the care of a competent physician.

Ulcers can be irritated by not allowing enough time between eating and the time you lie down to go to sleep. Because all of your body functions slow down while you're sleeping, the stomach does not digest food quickly, and excessive acid is produced. To avoid irritating ulcers, doctors recommend that a person should not eat for two to three hours before going to sleep.

People suffering with ulcers were formerly encouraged to drink milk to "coat" their stomachs before eating or going to bed. However, in the last few years, researchers have discovered that milk stimulates acid production, so it should be avoided by people with ulcers.

A study involving almost 200 patients in four countries showed that Maalox® Therapeutic Concentrate, taken twice daily, reduces recurrences of duodenal ulcers. Daily Maalox® was just two percent less effective than the prescription drug Tagamet®, which is widely prescribed to prevent recurring ulcers. Since Maalox® has few side effects and is available at much less cost than Tagamet®, this study could change ulcer treatment. The study results were presented at a recent meeting of the American College of Gastroenterology, as reported in <u>USA</u> <u>Today</u>.

Urination, Painful

Some women complain of painful urination even when there is no infection present. Now doctors are finding that women who frequently use soap directly on, or in, the vaginal area often suffer from painful urination (<u>The</u> <u>Lancet</u>). Doctors are starting to recommend eliminating the use of soap, talcum powder and colored or perfumed toilet paper in the vaginal area.

Urinary Incontinence

Urinary leakage or "shrinking bladders" becomes more common as we grow older, but some kinds of leakage can be cured by simple exercises. Leakage caused by simple movements like laughing, sneezing or sudden movement is called "stress incontinence". Incontinence can be annoying and embarrassing. It can become so bad that the person cannot sleep through the night. In some cases, these problems are caused by a weak pelvic muscle, called the pubococcygeus or PC muscle, and can be cured by simple exercises.

PC exercises, sometimes called "Kegel" exercises,

were started in 1952 by Arnold Kegel, a gynecologist from the University of Southern California. He started the exercises as part of the recovery program from bladder surgery. Soon, Dr. Kegel discovered that the exercises alone often prevented the need for bladder surgery.

Now, research has shown that by exercising the muscles for just 15 minutes each day, many causes of urinary incontinence, urinary tract infections, and menstrual cramps can be reduced or cured. As a pleasant side effect, PC exercises increase the likelihood of a woman experiencing orgasm during intercourse, and increase sexual endurance for men by 50%, according to Dr. William E. Hartman and Marilyn Fithian at the Center for Marital and Sexual Studies in Long Beach, California.

PC EXERCISES — The most important thing about starting PC exercises is to locate and isolate the correct muscle. To locate the muscle, sit on the toilet and open your legs as far as possible. Try to stop the flow of urine by contracting the PC muscle. Relax the muscle, letting the urine flow, then stop and start the flow. In both men and women, the muscle that stops and starts the flow, is the pubococcygeus or PC muscle. Once you know what using the muscle feels like, you can exercise it when you are not urinating. This is the muscle that you want to exercise for fifteen minutes each day.

Four main exercises are recommended: "flicks"

— contract and release the PC muscle to the time of a fast beat, like your heartbeat; "holds" — hold the PC muscle as tight as possible for 10 seconds, then release, then repeat; "bear downs" — bear down for three seconds, then release; "gradual holds" — gradually, to a slow count of ten, contract the PC muscle, then to another count of ten, slowly relax it. You may need to start slowly and build up to 15 minutes a day. Even though these exercises sound simple, they often make the difference between good bladder control and lack of control.

As well as doing the Kegel exercises, older people with urinary incontinence should remember to empty their bladders regularly, even if they don't feel the urge to do so. By emptying the bladder, they will avoid putting unnecessary pressure on it, which can cause lack of control.

Urinary Tract Infections

Urinary tract infections should be treated under a physician's care and advice.

Cranberry juice may be helpful in treating urinary tract infections, according to a study by Anthony E. Sobota published in The Journal of Urology. The research discovered that within one to three hours after people drink cranberry juice, they have an "anti-cling" substance present in the urinary tract. This substance makes it difficult for bacteria to cling to the walls of the urinary tract or to the bladder. Since the bacteria are not able to stay in the tract, the cranberry juice promotes faster relief from the infection. The "anti-cling" factor in the cranberry juice seems to work for up to 15 hours. Cranberry juice can often be used with other forms of treatment.

If you suffer from urinary tract infections, do not use bubble bath. According to the U.S. Food and Drug Administration, "Excessive use (of bubble bath) or prolonged exposure may cause irritation to skin and urinary tract. Discontinue use if rash, redness or itching occurs."

In some cases, urinary tract infections are caused by a weak pelvic muscle, called the pubococcygeus or PC muscle, and can be cured by simple exercises. Research has shown that by exercising the muscles for just 15 minutes each day urinary incontinence, urinary tract infections, and menstrual cramps can be reduced or cured. For complete information on how to perform these simple exercises, please see: **PC EXERCISES** — under **Urinary Incontinence**.

Vaginitis

Vaginitis is an inflammation of the vagina which may be caused by an infection. Several natural remedies have been suggested as ways to prevent or cure vaginitis, but none has actually been proven or disproven. Wearing cotton underpants, because they "breathe" better than synthetic underpants has been recommended by some people. Douching is sometimes recommended, but many doctors now feel that douching interrupts the normal cleansing processes of the body and may do more harm than good. Putting yogurt into the vagina has been suggested, since the bacteria in yogurt are similar to the beneficial bacteria normally found in the vagina. This treatment has not been proven to be effective against vaginitis.

Varicose Veins

Varicose veins can be prevented or reduced by simple, natural changes in your lifestyle. Wear support hose, raise or elevate the legs frequently, eat a diet rich in fiber, don't cross your legs, try not to stand or sit for long periods of time, get plenty of exercise, especially exercise that uses the legs, like walking, jogging, swimming, dancing or cycling. If you are overweight, lose weight, avoid wearing tight shoes or boots and consider learning and practicing foot massage.

Low-fiber diets that cause pressure on the veins from a large fecal mass in the abdomen are the chief cause of varicose veins. Diets containing plenty of bran or other sources of fiber are a good remedy.

Crossing the legs may be another reason that women suffer from varicose veins and blood clots. Crossing the legs, especially at the thighs, impairs the flow of blood in the veins and arteries of the legs. When varicose veins or vascular disease is present, slower blood flow may cause formation of blood clots. Clots can be deadly if they move to the lungs, heart or brain. Crossing your legs at the ankles is not as harmful as crossing them at the thighs, but should also be avoided if possible.

Sitting for long periods of time, while recuperating, traveling or working, can also lead to formation of varicose veins and blood clots. Be sure to get up and walk around at least once every two hours to renew the circulation to your legs and feet. Rotate your feet and ankles whenever possible to improve circulation.

If immediate family members have varicose veins, be especially careful to follow these instructions and try to prevent varicose veins from occurring, since a tendency towards varicose veins can be inherited.

Warts

Warts are caused by viruses in the skin. They usually affect teenagers, but they can affect anyone. There are many different kinds of warts; some appear as bumps on the hands and face and another common variety, plantar warts, are usually located on the soles of the feet.

Home remedies for regular warts have many variations, including putting dandelion juice, cod-liver oil, vitamin E or aloe on the warts. Some people file down the warts with an emery board or cover them with band-aids until they become brittle. Then they apply aloe juice or other moisturizer and file them again. Repeat the filing and moisturizing until the warts disappear. Since warts are caused by a virus, it is difficult to tell whether the "remedy" caused the warts to go away or if they went away on their own.

Dabbing on strong solutions of salicylic acid in ether, sold over-the-counter, to burn off the warts is the most effective home treatment.

Because plantar warts are on the bottom of the feet and bear the body's weight, they grow into the foot, rather than into an outward bump like most other warts. The inward growth develops a core and thick layer of callus around it. They can be very painful. Some people catch plantar warts from walking barefoot in public showers, locker rooms, hotel rooms or around swimming pools. Other people seem immune to the wart virus.

Home treatment for plantar warts means helping to remove the pressure from the wart. Pad the area around the wart with felt or moleskin. This will relieve the strain of the wart supporting the body's weight and should help reduce the pain.

Remove all dead skin from the plantar wart, then soak the whole affected foot in hot water (as hot as you can take it — about 118°F) for 15 minutes daily. After two weeks of these hot daily baths, it seems as if the plantar virus is beaten, and the warts often disappear completely.

Water Retention: See Fluid Retention

Weight Loss

A recent study published in <u>Postgraduate</u> <u>Medicine</u> (79: 4: 352) showed that people could lose weight by changing the time of day that they eat.

By altering their food intake to the morning and noon meals, with just a light afternoon snack, almost 600 people lost between 5 - 10 pounds each a month. The participants did not change the amount of food they ate, just the time of day it was eaten. They could not go to sleep within eight hours of their last meal. Although these are just preliminary results from a study at Tulane University, changing the time of daily eating may be a worthwhile method for people trying to lose weight.

Proper nutrition, combined with regular exercise, will help you lose weight and improve your overall health. A recent report by the U.S. Health and Human Services explained that most obesity is caused by underexercising rather than overeating. Therefore, cutting back on high-fat diets while increasing the amount of daily exercise is a key to overcoming obesity.

Sports physicians are now recommending exercise that includes use of both the legs and the arms, according to <u>Physician</u> <u>and</u> <u>Sports</u> <u>Medicine</u> (14:5, 181). Window washers, farmers and orchestra conductors, all people that use their arms daily, seem to have an increased life expectancy. Sports physicians recommend using the arms for a complete exercise program. The best workouts for the whole body are swimming, cross-country skiing or using a rowing machine, says the article.

Wrinkles

To prevent wrinkles, we should watch the way we speak and the way we sleep, says Samuel Stegman, a dermatologist from San Francisco. When talking we often frown, tighten our lips and make other faces that help create wrinkles, Stegman says. He suggests placing a mirror by your telephone to see how you move your face, so you can develop better facial control. Pushing your head into your pillow when you sleep can cause wrinkles, too. Some wrinkles and skin creases are directly related to how people sleep, according to Stegman. To help prevent wrinkles, try to avoid pushing your head and face into your pillow or mattresses.

Yeast Infections

Thousands of women suffer from yeast infections, which often occur in the vagina and cause itching, swelling, burning, painful urination, soreness and a white discharge.

There are not any good natural cures once the infection is present, but there are several ways to avoid aggravating the infection, according to researcher Dr. Marjorie Crandall. Don't use soaps, talcum powder, perfumed or colored toilet paper, douches, chlorinated water or spermicides. Also, wearing panty-hose or tight jeans may be aggravating since they can provide the proper conditions for the infection to grow. People with yeast infections should also avoid eating any food containing yeast such as breads, cheese, beer or wine. Sugar intake should also be severely limited, since sugar can also promote the growing conditions for the infection.

In Closing

The natural healing secrets in this book are based on medical reports, but don't overlook the supernatural healing power of God. God is our Creator and the Master Physician. If you put your faith and trust in God, by following Jesus Christ, your prayers for healing will be answered according to God's will.

If you would like to know more about how to know God and have eternal life through a personal relationship with Jesus Christ, please write to: FC&A, Dept JC 87, 103 Clover Green, Peachtree City, Georgia, 30269. We believe getting to know God better will change your life!

Bibliography

The Aging Eye: Facts on Eye Care for Older Persons. National Society to Prevent Blindness. New York, NY. 1986.

American Health. T. George Harris, editor. American Health Partners, New York, NY 1986.

Bricklin, Mark. *Mailbag of Natural Remedies*. Rodale Press, Emmaus, PA. 1982.

Brody, Jane. *"185 Nutrition Tips for 1985"* Family Circle. January 15, 1985.

Cawood, Frank W. and Janice McCall Failes. *Hidden Health Secrets*. FC&A Publishing, Peachtree City, GA. 1986.

Cawood, Frank W. and Rita Warmack. *Arteries Cleaned Out Naturally*. FC&A Publishing, Peachtree City, GA. 1986

Cawood, Frank W. *Vitamin Side Effects Revealed*. FC&A Publishing, Peachtree City, GA. 1986

Ellis, Jeffrey W., M.D. and Editors of Consumer Guide®. *Medical Symptoms and Treatments*. Publications International, Skokie, IL. 1983.

Healthline. — September 1986. Paul M. Insel, Ph.D. Editor. Robert A. McNeil Foundation Publishing, Menlo Park, CA. 1986.

Healthwise. Alexander Grant, M.D., editor. Alexander Grant, M.D. and Associates, Indianapolis, IN. 1986.

Kotecki, Nancy. *Nancy's No Nonsense Tips.* Regal Greetings and Gifts, Toronto, Ontario, Canada. 1983.

Mayo Clinic Health Letter. Joseph M. Kiely, M.D., editor. Mayo Foundation, Rochester, MN. 1986.

Obesity and Your Health. American College of Obstetricians and Gynecologists. Washington, DC 1986.

The Prevention® Natural Medicine Cabinet. editors of Prevention® Magazine. Rodale Press, Inc. Emmaus, PA. 1986.

Rosenfeld, Dr. Isadore. *Modern Prevention: The New Medicine.* Simon & Schuster, Inc. New York, NY. 1986.

Sanes-Miller, Carol H., editor. *Family Medical and Health Guide.* Publications International. Skokie, IL. 1985.

Sore Throats: Causes and Cures. American Academy of Otolaryngology — Head and Neck Surgery, Inc. Washington, DC 1986.

Smoking and Women. American College of Obstetricians and Gynecologists. Washington, DC 1986.

Wade, Carlson. *Natural Folk Remedies.* Globe Mini Mags, 1986.

UCLA Health Insights. Gary Gitnick, M.D., editor. Medcom, Inc. Garden Grove, CA. 1986.

"He Died With Arteries Like A Baby"

Researchers Discover Evidence That The Human Body Has Its Own Natural System That Helps Keep The Arteries Clean

(Atlanta, GA)

Can your arteries be cleaned out naturally? That's what many doctors are asking themselves after an autopsy of a famous nutrition expert who committed suicide.

Can The Body Keep Its Arteries Clean?

What interests the doctors is that the "free from artery disease" theory of the nutrition expert may be proven by his death! The doctor who performed the autopsy was, in his own words "amazed to find no evidence of coronary artery disease in a man of his age (69)". He said that the nutrition expert had "arteries like a baby". What's even more amazing is that the nutrition expert was diagnosed as actually having coronary artery disease 30 years earlier when he was 39 years old.

The nutrition expert put himself on a special program to fight coronary artery disease. You'll learn about it in a new $9.95 book for the general public, *"Arteries Cleaned Out Naturally"*.

It reveals a startling new discovery by medical researchers. They say they have discovered evidence that the human body has its own natural system that helps keep the arteries clean.

Case studies like this may be atypical. There is no proof that already narrowed or clogged arteries will open up when we start to do things which might help the body's natural cleansing process.

The Amazing Story of LDL's and HDL's

You'll learn about the new scientific discovery that the human body seems to have its own natural system which helps keep the arteries clean.

You'll learn about how LDL molecules seem to carry cholesterol into the walls of coronary arteries and lead to heart and artery disease. You'll also learn about how other molecules, HDL's, seem to play a part in the body's natural cleansing system.

The recent discoveries about HDL's are important because researchers think that most coronary artery disease is avoidable.

What *"Arteries Cleaned Out Naturally"* Reveals

- The amazing story of HDL's.
- Four different types of heart and artery disease explained in easy-to-understand language
- Why hardening of the arteries and high blood pressure may be higher now than years ago
- Vitamins and minerals . . . can they help prevent artery disease?
- Exercise . . . one type that's harmful, another type that helps
- Why some people get heart attacks even though they're health conscious
- Heart surgery . . . when it's likely not to help . . . when relief may be obtained by other means
- Why some fat people don't suffer from artery disease
- Low-fat diets, are they helpful?
- Relaxation training . . . is it for you?
- Why foot problems are associated with high rates of heart attack
- Does smoking really cause heart attacks?
- Does salt cause high blood pressure?
- How to add 10 years to your life

Free With Order

Order now and we will send you absolutely free, our newsletter, *"Health News"*.

You must cut out and return this notice with your order. Copies will not be accepted!

Order *"Arteries Cleaned Out Naturally"* now! Tear out and return this notice with your name and address and a check for $9.95 + $2.00 shipping and handling to our following address: FC&A, Dept. XSZ-3, 103 Clover Green, Peachtree City, GA 30269.

Save! Return this notice with $19.90 + $2.00 for two books. (No extra shipping and handling charges.)

You also get an unconditional money-back guarantee. If you're not 100% satisfied for any reason, any time, send *"Arteries Cleaned Out Naturally"* back and we will cheerfully refund your purchase price, no questions asked, but keep your free newsletter. ©FC&A 1987

"High Blood Pressure Lowered Naturally"

(Atlanta, GA)

FC&A, a nearby Peachtree City, Georgia medical publisher, announced today the release of a new $3.99 research report for the general public, *"High Blood Pressure Lowered Naturally"*.

It reveals a startling new discovery at a world famous medical center: the reversal of high blood pressure without prescription drugs! A discovery unknown to most people.

What Your Doctor Doesn't Tell You

A recent U.S. Government survey revealed that most doctors don't tell their patients about the possible side effects of drugs they prescribe. Tell your doctor if you have any possible side effects given in this research report for high blood pressure drugs.

The Good Effects Of Lowering High Blood Pressure

You or those you love may take prescription drugs to lower blood pressure, relieve pain, reduce fluid buildup, regulate heartbeat or prevent strokes and heart attacks.

Dangerous Side Effects Of High Blood Pressure Drugs

Unfortunately, high blood pressure drugs can cause miserable side effects like headaches, poor appetite, upset stomach, dry mouth, diarrhea, stuffy nose, dizziness, tingling or numbness in the hands or feet.

Now Blood Pressure Can Be Lowered Without Drugs

Recently, a university study has proven that most cases of high blood pressure can be lowered without drugs. 85.3% of patients with high blood pressure were able to quit taking drugs.

Amazingly, their blood pressure remained lower than when they were on drugs. Cholesterol levels also dropped 26%. The doctor in charge said of this program, "You lose your tiredness. You feel much more active. You have a general feeling of well being."

How Did They Do It?

How did the hundreds of people in this study free themselves from the miserable side effects of drugs—drugs they thought they would have to take for the rest of their lives?

Why are medical doctors saying that the findings are "very exciting" and that many patients have "a new lease on life".

These questions are all answered in a new research report, *"High Blood Pressure Lowered Naturally"*. You can order it by returning this notice and $3.99 to the address below.

Easy To Read

Facts about lowering blood pressure without drugs are listed in 10 easy-to-understand sections. You'll learn about the latest research in nutrition. How the presence or absence of 4 minerals and 4 other nutrients in your food and water can dramatically change your blood pressure. How poisons in the environment can make blood pressure skyrocket! How relaxation training can help. Why blood pressure medicine is overprescribed.

FREE With Order

Order *"High Blood Pressure Lowered Naturally"* now and we will send you FREE, our newsletter, *Health News.*

You must cut out and return this notice with your order. Copies will not be accepted!

Order now! Tear out and return this notice with your name and address and a check for $3.99 + $2.00 shipping and handling to our following address: FC&A, Dept. 4SZ-3, 103 Clover Green, Peachtree City, GA 30269.

Save! Return this notice with $7.98 + $2.00 for two books. (No extra shipping and handling charges.)

There's a no-time limit guarantee of satisfaction or your money back.

©FC&A, 1987.